JN086940

ライフサイエンスのための英語

のための 英語

English for Life Sciences
II. Presentations

II. プレゼンテーション編

萩原明子
内藤麻緒 編著
小林　薫

東京化学同人

序

　私たちが思いを伝える手段はたくさんありますが，そのなかでも口頭で直接相手に伝えることの重要性を 2020 年から始まったパンデミックにより実感した方も多いのではないでしょうか．書き言葉では十分に表すことができないものでも，口頭では聴き手の反応を確認しながら，内容を調整しつつ，その場で適切な言葉を選び伝えることができるからです．パンデミックのため，対面での情報交換の機会が制限され，コミュニケーションがオンラインになり，2 年を経てわかったことは，私たちはまだオンラインだけでは思う存分意見の交換を行うことができない，ということでした．オンラインの便利なツールを用いれば確かに授業は成立します．教室で講義を聞くのと，自宅にいながらオンラインで参加するのとでは学ぶ内容に変わりはないかも知れません．でも，講義と講義の間に教室を移動する途中で先生や友達と話したり，講義のあとで質問をしに教卓に行ったり，宿題が間に合わなくなったことを伝えに行ったり，といった日常のコミュニケーションが，実は学びを促進させてきたのだと実感しました．

　この教科書は，調べたことやわかったことを英語で聴き手に伝える方法（プレゼンテーション）を学ぶためのツールです．プレゼンテーションには参加者が共通に用いるスタイルや情報交換の決まり事のようなものがあります．コンピュータ用語ではプロトコルといいますが，情報を送り出す側と受取る側が同じ決まり事（プロトコル）に従うことで情報のやり取りを円滑にするものです．学術分野の新たな知見を他の研究者に伝えるプレゼンテーションにもそのような決まり事があります．ルールとは違って義務的なものではなく，分野や場所によっても変わるものなので，多くの場合「場数をふむ」ことによって覚えていくものでした．しかし，対面の学術交流の場が限られてしまった今，体験して学ぶということが以前よりも難しくなっています．こんな状況だからこそ，プレゼンテーションに関する基本的な事柄を体系的に学び，練習しておくことが重要なのです．そうすれば，実践の場で，発表する内容にもっと多くの時間を割くことができ，ゆとりをもって準備できるようになるでしょう．

　知らない人の前で，それも英語で考えを伝えることは簡単ではありません．しかし，この本を見て，やってみようという気になれたら，発表の準備の半分は終わったようなものです．この本では，簡単な例を用いることによって自然科学をテーマにしたプレゼンテーションの基本（スライドの作り方や話し方など）が学べるようになっています．大学生や大学院生だけでなく実験が大好きな中学生や高校生にも使っていただければと著者一同願っております．

　　2023 年 2 月

編 者 一 同

編　　集

萩　原　明　子　　東京薬科大学生命科学部 教授，Ph.D.
内　藤　麻　緒　　聖マリアンナ医科大学医学部 准教授，M.A.
小　林　　薫　　東京農業大学生命科学部 教授，Ph.D.

執　　筆

上　原　　岳　　専修大学大学院文学研究科博士後期課程，修士(文学)［付録 A～E］
小　林　　薫　　東京農業大学生命科学部 教授，Ph.D.［Unit 2～Unit 6］
小　村　桐　子　　東京薬科大学生命科学部 客員准教授，Ph.D.［Unit 1］
内　藤　麻　緒　　聖マリアンナ医科大学医学部 准教授，M.A.［Unit 2～Unit 6］
萩　原　明　子　　東京薬科大学生命科学部 教授，Ph.D.［Unit 2～Unit 6］
米　田　敦　子　　東京薬科大学生命科学部 講師，博士(理学)［Unit 2～Unit 6］
Germain Mesureur　　恵泉女学園大学人文学部 准教授，M.A.［Unit 2～Unit 5］

(五十音順，［　］内は執筆担当箇所)

動画ナレーション

米　田　敦　子　　東京薬科大学生命科学部 講師，博士(理学)
Germain Mesureur　　恵泉女学園大学人文学部 准教授，M.A.
Naomi K. Foster　　米国ウィスコンシン大学マディソン校

英語監修

Germain Mesureur　　恵泉女学園大学人文学部 准教授，M.A.

科学考証

米　田　敦　子　　東京薬科大学生命科学部 講師，博士(理学)

▶️ 動画のご利用方法

本書付属の"動画データ"を本書購入者本人に限り，下記の要領で取得できます．

1. 動画データの内容
内　容: video 1 ～ video 17
ファイル形式: MP4

2. 動画の再生方法
スマートフォンで QR コード*を読み取る方法と，パソコンで動画データをダウンロードする方法があります．
＊ QR コードは株式会社デンソーウェーブの登録商標です

2・1　QR コード*を読み取る（インターネットに接続した状態で）
お手持ちのスマートフォンで QR コード*を読み取ると，対応箇所の再生が始まります．

2・2　動画データをパソコンでダウンロードする
下記の手順，動作環境でダウンロードし，パソコンで再生してご利用ください．（購入者本人以外は使用できません．図書館での利用は館内での閲覧に限ります）

[ダウンロードの手順]
1) パソコンで東京化学同人のホームページにアクセスし，書名検索などにより，"ライフサイエンスのための英語 II. プレゼンテーション編"の書籍ページを表示させる．
2) 書籍ページよりダウンロードする動画を選ぶと，下の画面（Windows での一例）が表示されるので，ユーザー名およびパスワードを入力する．

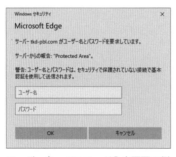

ユーザー名: **ELS2video**
パスワード: **mykuhkn**

[OK] を選択すると
ダウンロードが始まる

ユーザー名・パスワード入力画面の例

※ファイルは ZIP 形式で圧縮されています．解凍ソフトで解凍のうえ，ご利用ください．

目　　次

Unit 1

Introduction
プレゼンテーションとは

1・1 プレゼンテーションの定義，種類と目的

プレゼンテーションとは何かについて知る

Definition and purpose

A | **Definition**
What is a presentation?

 プレゼンテーションとは何か，まず英語で読んでみましょう．

Presentations are not just about telling someone about your story, thoughts, or ideas. A presentation conveys information from the presenter to the audience. This is a process of sharing, educating, and communicating your thoughts and ideas. Good presentations can impact people, communities, societies, and the world.

Terminology of a "presentation"

The word "presentation" has many meanings. The meaning of the verb "present" [prizént] used in the following examples can give you some clues.

- **Examples of the verb "present"**:
  - I present my research.
  - How do I present my research at a conference?

Definition of "presentation" — What are presentations?

- Your audience **learns** about [　　] from your presentation.
- Your audience **understands** [　　] from your presentation.
- Your presentation **describes** [　　] to your audience.
- Your presentation **identifies** [　　] to your audience.
- Your presentation **persuades** your audience about [　　].
- Your presentation **gives** something new to your audience.

In-person (face-to-face) and online presentations

Presentations are given in a variety of venues, situations and settings.

- **Examples of presentation situations and settings**:
  - Conference and meeting (In-person / online)
  - University admissions interview
  - Job interview

2　**Unit 1　Introduction**

今度プレゼンテーションをすることになったのですが，そもそもプレゼンテーションの定義とは何ですか？
学生

先生
英語では presentation といいますが，present【prizént】という動詞の名詞形です．何かを「提示する」とか「発表する」という意味です．"présent" と前にアクセントを置くと名詞では「贈り物」のことですし，形容詞なら「出席している」とか「現在の」という意味になる多くの意味をもつ言葉なので，誤解しないようにしましょう．

なるほど．そうすると，「発表すること」という意味で，発表する側である話し手と，発表を聴く側である聴き手がいるということですね．

それだけではありません．プレゼンテーションは，聴き手に自分の考えやストーリーを話して聴いてもらうだけではないのです．聴き手と知識や情報を共有することによるコミュニケーションなのです．いいプレゼンテーションは，聴き手だけでなく，コミュニティや社会にまで影響を及ぼす力をもっています．

えーっ！学校ではクラスで発表するプレゼンテーションしかやったことがないので知りませんでした．プレゼンテーションってそんなにディープなんですね．ってことは，学校以外の会社なんかでも行われるのですか？
学生

もちろん！ビジネスの世界でもよく行われます．むしろビジネスの現場で行うほうが一般的でしょう．IT 企業が新製品を発表するために行うプレゼンテーションなどは，特によく知られていますね．

そっかー．そういえば，入試や就職試験の面接でプレゼンテーションが課される場合も増えてますよね？

そうですね．今では，研究や教育の場や企業の就職試験でも積極的にプレゼンテーションが行われるようになりました．プレゼンテーションが活用されるさまざまな場面について知っておくことが，プレゼンテーションの準備をするのに役立ちますよ．

ポイント プレゼンテーションとは
聴き手に，
- ○○について学んでもらうこと
- ○○を知ってもらうこと
- ○○を理解してもらうこと
- ○○を説明すること
- ○○に関して相手を説得すること
- ○○について期待させること
- ○○について共有すること
- ○○を指摘すること
- ○○のきっかけをつくること

ポイント プレゼンテーションがよく行われる場面
- 小中高，大学などの教育の場
- 入学試験の面接の場
- 大学や企業などの研究の場
- 就職活動の面接の場
- カンファレンスなどの会議の場
- ビジネスやセールスなどの営業の場
- 仮想現実やオンラインコミュニティ

［人物アイコンのイラスト：©miniwide/shutterstock.com］

プレゼンテーションの目的について，英語で読んでみましょう．

Participants / Attendees

- **A conference presenter**: A person who gives a presentation and officially provides information to an individual or group, or a person who provides information for the general public.
- **A conference audience**: A person who listens to a presenter, understands the presentation, is encouraged to take actions.

Examples of presentation purpose

1）To inform

A presenter provides information to an audience or compares it with information that the audience may already have.

2）To persuade

- A presenter influences or changes the attitudes and beliefs of the audience.
- A presenter encourages the audience to take certain levels of action.
- A presenter persuades the audience by using concrete examples.

3）To interact /communicate

- A presenter meets and finds the audience who is interested in their presentation.
- A presenter meets and finds the audience who are or may be encouraged by their presentation.
- A presenter finds and exchanges information with the audience they want to discuss about the presentation.

Importance of presentation skills

Great presentations can affect people, solve problems, and change the world. It is important to improve presentation skills for students to develop professionalism and self-confidence. Presentation skills also help students increase future opportunities, such as college admissions and careers.

では，プレゼンテーションの基本的な目的って何ですか？

 個々のプレゼンテーションには特定の目的がありますが，一般的には，相手に特定の情報を伝え，理解してもらい，相手の行動変容を促すことです．

行動変容？ 要するに聴き手が，新しく得た情報に直接影響を受けて何かをするということですよね？

 そのとおり！セールスなど営業のプレゼンテーションを見たあとに，その商品を購入したら直接的な行動だとわかりますが，それだけではありません．たとえば科学研究のプレゼンテーションに触発されて，新しい研究方法を思いつけば，それもまた行動変容です．あるいは，よい研究の成果を効果的に伝えると，高い評価を得ることができ，受賞や研究費の獲得，それから人脈の形成にもつながります．

めちゃくちゃディープですね．聴き手に影響を与えるだけでなく，プレゼンターの将来もプレゼンテーションしだいで変わる可能性があるということですね．

 そうです．いいプレゼンテーションをするには，プレゼンテーションスキルを習得しておくことが重要です．

プレゼンテーションスキルを身につけるのは，研究者やビジネス界の方だけでなく，学生の私たちにとっても重要なんですね．では，効果的なプレゼンテーションとはどんなものですか？

 そうですね … やはり，情報共有が最もスムーズに行われるプレゼンテーションが効果的なプレゼンテーションだといえるでしょう．

そっかぁ．プレゼンテーションの目的にかなっていないと的外れなものなってしまいますね．

ポイント プレゼンテーションの目的
- 聴き手と新しい情報を共有すること
- 聴き手の行動変容を促すこと
- 聴き手について知ること
- 聴き手とネットワーキングすること

Tips 学会やカンファレンスに参加登録し，出席したりプレゼンテーションをしたり，または両方をする人たちのことを "attendees" といったりします．これは，「参加する」attend の動詞からきています．

Tips プレゼンテーション力を鍛える日々のトレーニング方法
身体を鍛えるために毎日エクササイズをするのと同じように，プレゼンテーション力を鍛える日々のトレーニングもしましょう．
おすすめのトレーニング：
- 日常会話を聞き取りやすい声で話す
- 情報を整理してシンプルにまとめる（ロジカルシンキング）
- 自分の癖や先入観を認識する（クリティカルシンキング）
- Twitter のように文字制限をして，今の状況や考えを相手に簡潔に説明する
- 制限時間内に固有名詞をキーワードやジェスチャーで説明するゲーム（Heads Up！などの連想ゲームのスマホアプリがおすすめ）
- TED Talks などのプレゼンテーション動画を YouTube チャンネルで視聴する

C   Presentation types and situations
What are the different types of presentations?

  プレゼンテーションの種類について英語で読んでみましょう.

There are several different types of presentations :

1) Informative presentations

   e.g., Academic lectures, research presentations, informative speeches

2) Instructive presentations

   e.g., Workshops, students orientations, webinars, employee training sessions

3) Persuasive presentations

   e.g., Research competitions, elevator pitches, sales pitches, investor pitches, business plans, sales proposals, event proposals, self-introductions

4) Motivational presentations

   e.g., Keynotes, storytelling, histories and overviews of organizations

5) Decision-making presentations

   e.g., A Company's business meetings, new product marketing meetings, negotiation meetings, face covering government's policy meetings, institutional board meetings

6) Progress presentations

   e.g., Weekly/Monthly reports, research progress reports, team stand up presentations

7) Other : Free style

   e.g., Music and performing arts

This textbook mainly discusses **informative presentations**. An informative presentation is a type of presentation to present facts and research findings to an audience. The presentation is logical and has an outline. This is often seen within educational settings, such as classrooms, research seminars, and academic conferences. When the presenter makes an informative presentation, the presentation needs to be enlightening and must be communicated so that the audience can understand the particular topic.

Instructive presentations are very similar to informative presentations. However, presenters can inform the audience of more than facts and findings. When the presenter makes an instructive presentation, the presenter can specify learning goals and objectives that can be taught and trained to the audiences to learn new skills.

プレゼンテーションにはどんな種類がありますか？

 プレゼンテーションの目的や形式によって，さまざまな種類があります．たとえば，レクチャーや研究セミナーのようなアカデミックなもの，それからビジネスの現場で企画や提案をするようなものがあります．

そんなに多くの種類があるのですね．では，どんな場面で，実際にプレゼンテーションをするのですか？

 いろいろな種類のプレゼンテーションがあるように，日常でも，学校でも，ビジネスでも，さまざまな場面が想定されます．

つまり，プレゼンテーションの種類や場面によって対象も変わってきますね？

 そのとおり！プレゼンテーションの準備をする前に，聴き手が誰かまず知っておくことがとても重要です．誰を対象に情報を伝えるかを明確にしなければなりません．

じゃあ，プレゼンテーションの聴き手についてあらかじめ調べておかなくてはいけませんね．

 そうです．聴き手が何について興味があるかも十分に考えて準備をしなければなりません．聴き手の立場にたって，行動変容を促すような情報の伝え方を工夫しましょう．

プレゼンテーションの種類，対象，場面を知っておくことが，プレゼンテーションの準備なのですね．

- レクチャー
- イベント・企画の提案
- 新製品の発表
- 研究成果の報告
- スピーチ
- ピッチ*1（売り込み）
- 面接の自己PR

*1 ピッチとは，プレゼンテーションにおいて，「短い時間内に，聴き手にわかりやすく，心を打つ提案をすること」を意味します．ビジネスの世界で起業（start up）をするときに製品やアイディアを売込むための短いスピーチとして使われています．エレベーターの中のような短い時間で商品や自分自身を売込むエレベーターピッチ，営業マンのセールスピッチなどがあります．

ポイント さまざまなプレゼンテーションの場面

- アカデミック（授業内・研究室）
- 学会・研究会（カンファレンス/コンファレンス）
- 講演会（フォーラム・シンポジウム・パネル討議）
- 研修会（セミナー）
- ワークショップ
- 企画・提案会議
- ウェビナー*2・オンライン会議
- ピッチコンテスト
- リサーチコンペ
- 学校や企業説明会
- 入学試験や就職試験
- 成果報告会

*2 ウェビナー（Webinar）とは，Web＋Seminar のことで，オンラインで Web 会議システムを利用して行われるセミナーのこと．

目的，種類，場面，対象，媒体，ツール，服装（身だしなみ）を確認する

Pre-planning

A　**Defining and understanding your audience**
Who is your audience for the presentation?

 事前に準備すべきことについて英語で読んでみましょう．

It is very important to know who your audience is in the presentation. If you can define your audience, you can prepare your presentation effectively. If you know and understand your audience, you can deliver your presentation well. Therefore, defining and understanding your audience is part of an important pre-planning process. The audience for a presentation depends on the type and context of the presentation. Let's think about who the audience is for your presentation. It is important to know the objective of the presentation. For example, is your audience familiar with your research topic? What does the audience expect from your presentation?

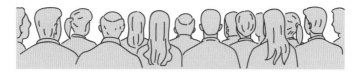

Different types of audiences
[© jesadaphorn/shutterstock.com]

Examples of different types of presentation audiences：

1）Academic audiences

e.g., Instructors, classmates, research lab members, collegiate teams, students clubs

2）Business audiences

e.g., Marketing and sales customers, investors, judges

3）Experts

e.g., Panel of research experts, research foundations, corporate foundations

4）Attendees and participants

e.g., Webinar attendees, workshop attendees, event participants

5）Interviewers (c.f., university admissions / employment)

e.g., University admissions officers, professors / employers, human resources staff

---

プレゼンテーションを通して，話し手と聴き手の間で双方向のコミュニケーションをしているのですね．プレゼンテーションの対象を配慮することは，とても大切ですね．

 そのとおり！そのほか，聴き手が満足できるように，聴き手のニーズを分析しておくことは，事前準備において大事なプロセスの一つです．右下の表のように考えてみましょう．

では，プレゼンテーションの対象に適した，聴き手により正確な情報を伝えるにはどのようなツールや形式がありますか？

 いい質問ですね！プレゼンテーションの形式には，ポスターや口述があります．最近では，オンラインで行われることも多くあります．プレゼンテーションのツールは，形式に合わせて選ぶのがおすすめです．最もよく使われるのは，プレゼンテーションのためのソフトウェアで作成したスライドです．

事前に準備しなければならないことがたくさんあるんですね．一つひとつ確認をして準備をしておかないと，聴き手に届くいいプレゼンテーションにはなりませんね．

ポイント プレゼンテーションの対象にはさまざまなタイプがあります．以下はその例です．
1) 学校関係: 教員，クラスメイト，研究室のメンバー，部活メンバー
2) ビジネス: 新商品発表に興味のある消費者，ピッチコンテストの審査員，投資家
3) 専門家: 研究者（同じ専門分野，違う専門分野），研究支援をする公的機関，企業，財団など
4) 一般: 会議，ウェビナー，ワークショップなどのイベントの出席者・参加者
5) 企業や大学: 入学希望者，就職希望者，面接試験官

プレゼンテーションの対象がわかったら，次に対象が必要としていること，知りたいこと，興味のあることや物などを考えてみましょう．

プレゼンテーションの対象（聴き手）は…
1) 学校関係
・どんな知識や情報が必要ですか？
2) ビジネス
・どんな要望がありますか？
・どんな問題を抱えていますか？
・その原因や解決策について知りたいですか？
3) 専門家
・どのような背景知識をもっていますか？
・どのような知識が必要ですか？
4) 一般
・どんな課題を抱えていますか？
・またその原因は？
・どのようなことに興味がありますか？
・どのような状況や環境にありますか？
5) 企業や大学
・どのような学生（人材）を探していますか？
・どのような商品開発のアイディアを探していますか？

B Presentation formats, tools, and materials
What are presentation formats, tools, and materials/visual aids?

プレゼンテーションの形式に合ったツール選びについて英語で読んでみましょう.

The presenter should carefully choose the best presentation tools and materials (visual aids) for each presentation format and platform. Various presentation tools may be used. You need to know the format of your presentation. Most of the tools and materials are commonly used in both face-to-face (in-person) and online presentation platforms. Knowing about presentation tools can be very helpful in creating presentation slides. Examples of presentation tools include Microsoft PowerPoint, Keynote, Google Slides, Prezi, and Canva.

In-person and online presentations

Formats	Tools (in-person)	Tools (Online)	Materials/Visual Aids
Paper session (Oral presentation)	Slides Whiteboard Projector, PC, microphone	Slides screen share Interactive whiteboard Web conference systems	Handouts Audio, video Pictures, models
Panel session	Slides	Slides screen share, PC	Handouts
Poster session (Poster presentation)	Poster slides Easel Tri-fold display, poster	Slides screen share, PC Conference specified web-based formats Conference specified web portals Pre-recorded videos and presentations	Poster Handouts Business cards
Roundtable session	Tables, chairs	Web conference systems	Handouts
Symposium	Slides, microphone	Slides screen share, microphone	Handouts
Workshop	Slides	Slides screen share Web conference systems, breakout rooms	Handouts

Presentation attire
- ### What is presentation attire?
  It is important to choose proper and comfortable clothing so that you can look professional and feel confident. The style of clothing depends on the theme of the meeting, the community, and the style (in-person or online). For online presentations, you can also effectively choose virtual backgrounds and lights to make a good impression on your audiences.

- ### Examples:
  Tailored shirt, collared shirt, shirt dress with jacket, pant suit, pants / skirt and blouse, business-casual suit, business suit and tie

Business card
Business cards help presenters stay in touch with the audience. We recommend that you bring at least 100 business cards when you attend a conference.

プレゼンテーションツールや資料，メディア媒体（下表を参照）のほかにも，事前に準備しておいたほうがいいことがありますか？

いろいろありますが，服装（身だしなみ）があります．プレゼンテーションの会場，対象を配慮し，相手が気持ちよく発表を聞けるように気をつけたほうがいいでしょう．過剰にドレスアップをしたり，就職活動で着用するようなお決まりのスーツばかりを着る必要はありません．事前に服装（身だしなみ）のチェックをしておくと，プレゼンテーションの当日になっても慌てずにすみますね．

服装についてあまり考えていませんでした．プレゼンテーションの聴き手によい印象を与えることも大事ですね．

プレゼンテーションの時（Time），場所（Place），目的・シーン（Occasion）に沿って，フォーマルであるべきか，ビジネスカジュアルが適しているか，カジュアルなほうがいいかなども含めて服装を考えてみましょう．それから，顔の表情が明るく，しっかり見えるように気をつけ，清潔感があるほうがいいですね．

ポイント 服装（身だしなみ）チェックリスト

- TPO に沿った清潔感のある服，靴下，靴，かばんのコーディネート
- 顔がしっかり見える髪型や顔まわり
- 眼鏡，時計，アクセサリーは過度に装飾的でないもの

Tips バーチャル背景：オンラインプレゼンテーションでは，バーチャル背景やライト，カメラ，マイクなどを効果的に使い，プレゼンテーションを引き立て，相手にプロフェッショナルに見えるよう工夫しましょう．

名 刺：ソフトウェアで簡単に作成することができます．プレゼンテーション用に 100 枚くらい作成しておくと，聴き手と連絡先を交換し，ディスカッションを発展させるなど効果的に使えます．

対面とオンラインのプレゼンテーション

形 式	ツール（対面での開催）	ツール（オンライン開催）	効果的な補助資料
口頭発表	・発表スライド ・ホワイトボード ・プロジェクター，PC，マイク	・スライドの画面共有 ・電子黒板 ・Web 会議システム	・ハンドアウト ・オーディオ，ビデオ ・視覚的資料（写真・モデル）
パネル	発表スライド	スライドの画面共有，PC	ハンドアウト
ポスター発表[*1]	・ポスタースライド ・イーゼル ・3 つ折りディスプレイ，ポスターボード	・スライドの画面共有，PC ・学会指定の Web フォーマット ・学会指定の Web ポータル ・ブレイクアウトセッション	・ポスター ・ハンドアウト ・名 刺
ラウンドテーブル[*2]	テーブル，椅子	Web 会議システム	ハンドアウト
シンポジウム	・発表スライド ・Q＆Aマイク	・スライドの画面共有 ・Web 会議システム	・ハンドアウト ・フィードバック用アンケート
ワークショップ	発表スライド	・スライドの画面共有 ・ブレイクアウトセッション	ハンドアウト

*1　ポスター発表におけるプレゼンテーションについては，Unit 6 に詳しい説明があります．
*2　ラウンドテーブル（Roundtable session）は，トピックごとに丸形テーブルが複数設定されていて，各テーブルに参加者や発表者が集まって意見交換や情報共有を口頭で行う交流型プレゼンテーションです．

1・3 プレゼンテーションの準備
スライドやポスターをつくる

Preparation

A Brainstorming
What do you do as the first step?

 プレゼンテーションを準備するとき最初にすべきことについて英語で読んでみましょう.

Step 1 Brainstorming:

Brainstorming will make you think creatively about the "big picture" of your presentation. Writing down a list of your ideas is a good way to get started with brainstorming. It is very helpful to see a clear idea for your presentation. Please try to list the ideas that come to your mind. There are no bad ideas. All ideas are good ideas.

Let's try brainstorming!

  - What are the topics for your presentation?
  - What are your general ideas?
  - What are your main ideas?
  - What are your areas of interest?

After brainstorming, share your ideas with your friends and classmates. Then, take turns and discuss. Do not judge or criticize ideas but encourage everyone to speak up.

Creating concept and mind maps are also useful.

Step 2 Choosing design templates:

After brainstorming, you can think about which design is a good match for your presentation's main topic. Designing all the slides yourself is not easy. However, the presentation tools have many good design templates installed.

Do you know what a design template is?

Design templates are pre-made presentation design formats with a consistent appearance. Templates have useful layouts such as title and subtitle slides, title and content slides, and more. In addition, there are various themes and colors. You can explore all different types of design templates; choose the one that works best for your presentation and customize it. For example, you can insert a college logo or change the background color to the school color. Don't forget to resize the slides to fit with the projector or web conferencing system you'll be using. Thus, design templates make it easy to create your own slides.

では，さっそくプレゼンテーションの準備を始めましょう．

最初にいったい何を準備すればいいですか？

 まずは，プレゼンテーション全体のブレインストーミングをしましょう．

そもそも，ブレインストーミングって何ですか？

 ブレインストーミングとは，もともとは会議の参加者たちがたがいのアイディアを自由に出し合い，1人では考えられないような発想をするための手法です．ここでは，プレゼンテーションのテーマやトピックに沿ってあるだけのアイディアを書き起こす作業をさします．ブレインストーミングをすることによって，プレゼンテーション全体のイメージが湧いて，どのようにスライドやポスターのデザインをフォーマットするかを決定するのに大変役に立ちます．

なるほど！では，ブレインストーミングのアイディアを整理して，スライドのデザインはどのように決めればいいのでしょうか？

 とてもいい質問ですね．プレゼンテーションのスライドのデザインは，話す内容や聴き手に伝えたい情報のテーマやトピックに沿って決めるといいでしょう．

でも，自分でスライドやポスターをデザインするのは時間がめっちゃかかりそう … 何かいい方法を教えてください！

 デザインテンプレートを知っていますか？プレゼンテーションのソフトウェアにインストールされている既製のデザインテンプレートを活用すると簡単で便利です．スライドの背景やレイアウトがあらかじめ設定されているので，プレゼンテーションに沿って簡単にカタマイズをすることも可能です．たとえば，在籍する学校の名称やロゴ，スクールカラーなどに合わせてカスタマイズすることもよく見られます．

ポイント ブレインストーミングは，1950年代に考案された会議方式で，3名〜10名程度の集団で行うことが多いです．日本語では "ブレスト" と略されます．

参加者が守らなければならないブレインストーミングの4原則：
1) 他の参加者の意見を否定，批判してはいけない（批判厳禁）
2) 奇抜でも常識はずれなユニークなアイディアでも歓迎する
3) 質よりも量を重視する
4) 他の参加者の意見に自分の意見を加えて発展させる

バズセッション（Buzz session）：
Buzzはハチの羽音．バズセッションとは，6名前後の複数のグループでディスカッションをし，同時に発言をした際にハチがブンブン鳴っているように聞こえることからついた名称．バズセッションもブレインストーミングの1手法です．

ポイント ブレインストーミングのあとにすること：
- 出てきた多くのアイディアをすべて記録しましょう．スティッキーノート，スマホ，タブレットなどを使うと記録や共有がしやすいです．
- アイディアの整理をしましょう．最近では便利なアプリケーションツールがあります．(Slack, Google Documents, IdeaBoardz, Coggle, MindMup, Miro, Cacoo など)

Tips デザインテンプレート：最もよく使われるのは，PowerPointですが，最近ではデザイナーが作成したテンプレートが充実したCanvaのようなツールもあります．整理した情報を基に，どのテンプレートが一番適切か試してみましょう．

Presentation formats: Font type, color, and size
Which is the right font for the slides?

 プレゼンテーションスライドで用いるフォントについて英語で読んでみましょう.

Let's think which font to use! Choosing the right font types essentially affects the audience's level of understanding of the presentation. "Serif" and "Sans Serif" are the two main font types. The Sans Serif font type is primarily used for presentation slides.

Two major font types:
- Serif

  Serif font features a small extension or a small line (French: serif) at the end of the letter stroke. It is a decorative stroke similar to Japanese calligraphy art. The most common Serif font is Times New Roman. Other examples are Garamond and Georgia.

- Sans Serif (without Serif)

  Sans is French, which means "without." Sans Serif fonts have no decorative strokes. Using Sans Serif fonts on presentation slides make them look professional and easy to read. Examples include Arial, Calibri, Futura, Helvetica, and Tahoma. The recommended Japanese font types for presentation slides are Meiryo, MS Gothic, and MS P Gothic.

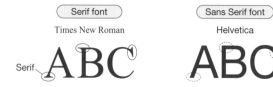

Font color and background color:

Which is better, high or low color contrast? Using high color contrast is better. If the background of the slide is a dark color, a bright or light color is suitable for the text. Blue, black, gray, brown, and white are standard, visually recognizable and professional on presentation slides. When choosing fonts and background colors, consider visually impaired people.

Font size:

Choosing the right font size is also important. Slides are a real-time presentation tool for communicating with your audiences. When choosing a font size, the presenter should consider the number of attendees in the audience, the size of the conference room, and the screen size (width and height). Additionally, the font size distinguishes the slide content to help the audience understand to recognize key points.

プレゼンテーションのスライドのフォントでは何に気を付ければいいですか？

書体，種類，色，大きさなどの選び方と使い方を配慮しなければなりません．フォントにはおもに2種類の書体（セリフ体とサンセリフ体）があります．種類を選択するときは，装飾のない字体（サンセリフ体）のほうがいいです．
また，スライドの文字が小さすぎると，聴き手が読んで内容を理解するのに時間がかってしまいます．

たとえば，プレゼンテーションのタイトルと内容を含むスライドでは，タイトルに使用するフォントは大きく，重要なポイントは色を変えたり，強調したりするなど，聴き手が見やすく理解しやすいフォントの色やサイズを選択することもとても大事です．

わかりました．フォントによってスライドの見やすさが違うのですね．「プレゼンテーションにはサンセリフ体！」覚えました．

セリフ体（Serif）とサンセリフ体（Sans Serif）：フォントには，以下のような書体によって2種類のフォントがあります．

装飾あり　　　　装飾なし

English English

セリフ体　　　　サンセリフ体

Serif は「筆記体」．書道のようにトメやハライのあるフォントです．Sans はフランス語で「〜なしで」という意味．つまり，サンセリフ体は，装飾のない書体であるということです．

日本語と英数字それぞれに，プレゼンテーションによく使われる定番フォントがあります（表A，表B）．同じフォントサイズでも，フォントの種類によって見やすさや文字の幅も違います．

表A　日本語用定番フォント

フォント名	書体見本（10 pt）
メイリオ	プレゼンテーション
游ゴシック	プレゼンテーション
MS ゴシック	プレゼンテーション
MS P ゴシック†	プレゼンテーション
HGP ゴシック†	プレゼンテーション

†フォント名に入っているPは，proportional の頭文字です．英数字・かな・カナによって文字幅が調整されており，さらに見やすくなっています．

表B　英数字用定番フォント

フォント名	書体見本（10 pt）
Times New Roman	Presentation 012345
Helvetica	Presentation 012345
Calibri	Presentation 012345
Tahoma	Presentation 012345
Arial	Presentation 012345
Egoe UI	Presentation 012345
Verdana	Presentation 012345
Garamond	Presentation 012345

C   The power of visualizing data: Charts, graphs, infographics, maps, and tables
What are the methods to visualize data for presentations?

 スライドに示すデータの視覚化について英語で読んでみましょう.

Data visualization, as the term implies, is a visual means of representing information based on data. Visualizing data enables your presentation to be more informative and helps the audience to understand your presentation more clearly. Examples of data visualization include charts, graphs, infographics (information + graphics), maps, and tables. When presenting your research methods and results, visualizing data is one of the most effective ways to inform the audience about important particulars and findings of your study.

Let's make good presentation slides and posters with effective data visualization!

Examples of data visualization:
- **Charts:** Area chart, bar chart, bubble chart, column chart, flow chart, line chart, matrix chart, pie chart, radar chart, scatter plot chart, stacked column chart (a.k.a. mekko chart), treemap chart
- **Graphs:** Bar graph (stacked bar graph), histogram, box and whisker plot, bullet graph, line graph, Venn diagram
- **Maps:** Geographically distribution map, flow map, heat map, dot map, point map, filled map
- **Tables:** Data table, pivot table
- **Other:** Digital dashboard, 2D and 3D modeling

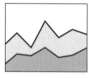
area chart

pie chart

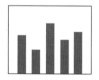
bar graph

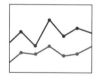
line graph

Tools and templates for visualizing data:
Creating and designing data visualization requires a certain level of skills. However, there are many data visualization tools for scientific presentations you can utilize. You can select the charts and graphs that are suitable for the results of your experiments.

Besides Microsoft Excel, Tableau, Microsoft Power BI and QlikView are data visualization tools that are designed to show interactively. Scientific researchers also use R and Python programming languages for data science and model simulation.

プレゼンテーションの聴き手にとって読みやすく，見やすいように視覚的な効果を考え，その手法を理解しておくことが大切なのですね．

そのとおり！視覚的な要素はフォントだけではありません．実験の方法や結果を，グラフや図，表などを使って視覚化します．聴き手がひと目で正確にデータを理解できるように，視覚的に効果のあるスライドやポスターを作成しましょう．

最近では，情報やデータを聴き手にわかりやすく表現し，グラフや図を用いて視覚的に伝える手段のことをインフォグラフィックといいます．

へぇー．そのほかにも，聴き手に情報をわかりやすく伝える手段がありますか？

もちろんです．音声や動画や写真などを活用すると，聴き手の知らない情報でもわかりやすく伝えることができ，理解を深め，満足させることにつながります．たとえばモデルシミュレーションでは，アニメーションが効果的に使われています．最近では，オンラインでの会議や学会が増えています．その場に相手がいなくても，臨場感を出す工夫をし，さまざまな視覚的な表現手法を取捨選択してスライドを作成しましょう．

OK！やってみます．では，データの視覚化を助けてくれるツールがありますか？

もちろん．データを視覚化し，プレゼンテーションのスライド上で表示するツールはいろいろあります．グラフやチャートを作るには Excel を使用することが多いですが，分野によってはプログラミング言語（R や Python）を使って出力したり，スライド上で表示する場合もあります．これらのスキルをつけるための勉強をするのも役に立つでしょう．

ポイント データビジュアライゼーション（**Data visualization**, データの視覚化）：スライドで研究の手法や結果を見せる方法は，グラフやチャート，表（Table）だけではありません．インフォグラフィック（Infographics）といって文字や絵やグラフなどの情報をまとめて視覚的に表現したり，ダッシュボード（Dashboard）のようにリアルタイムに更新されたデータをわかりやすく視覚化するツール（c.f., Tableau）もあります．統計ソフトなどで作成した表やグラフなどのデータソースに直接接続してダッシュボードを作成することが可能です．研究だけでなく企業のビジネスの現場でも多く使われています．

データビジュアライゼーションの例

図 （グラフ， チャート）	縦横棒グラフ，積み上げ縦横棒グラフ，ヒストグラム，箱ひげ図，ブレットグラフ，線グラフ，円グラフ，面グラフ，帯グラフ，メッコグラフ，散布図，バブルチャート，フローチャート，ベン図
マップ	地理的分布図，フローマップ，ヒートマップ，ポイントマップ，ドットマップ，塗りつぶしマップ
表（テーブル）	データテーブル，ピボットテーブル
その他	デジタルダッシュボード，2D・3D モデリング

1・4 スピーキング
話すことがらを整理する，効果的な話し方を知る

Speaking : Delivering your presentation

A **Organization and useful phrases**
How do you organize the content of your presentation?

 話すことがらの整理の重要性について英語で読んでみましょう．

You gathered all the information that you need to prepare for your presentation. What's next? Let's organize the content of your presentation, first. Organizing the presentation content helps in delivering your presentation for many reasons. Providing too much information can cause the audience to misunderstand the main idea of your presentation. Moreover, your presentation must be delivered within a certain timeframe, such as 10 minutes and 20 minutes. Structure your ideas by organizing the content, and you will have a clear outline of your presentation.

Let's try to compose and structure the entire presentation!
- How long is your presentation **time**?
- What is **significant** in your presentation?

プレゼンテーションの準備ができたら，今度は，実際に話すことがらを整理しましょう．

えーっ！どうして話すことがらを整理するのですか？たくさん話したいことがあるのですが…

 プレゼンテーションで話すことがらを整理するのには，理由がいくつかあります．スライドやポスターにのせる知識や情報が，必ずしも聴き手にとって必要ではないかもしれません．聴き手に配慮し，あらかじめ共有する情報を整理し，何を伝えたいのか重要なポイントがわかるようにしておいたほうがいいですね．

確かに！一方的に多くの情報を伝えても，聴き手にとってはまったくわからなかったり，つまらなかったり，価値がないものになってしまうかもしれませんね．では，話すことがらを整理するには，どのような手順ですればいいのでしょうか？

 まず，プレゼンテーション全体の構成を考えましょう．プレゼンテーション全体の流れがイメージできますよ．そうすれば，実際の発表のアウトラインを作成することができますね．

ほかに注意することはありますか？

 プレゼンテーションの制限時間を考えることです．時間内に重要なポイントをおさえて情報を共有するように気をつけましょう．

では，何かキーフレーズやキーワードも決めておいたほうがいいですよね．

 よく気がつきましたね！定型フレーズ（次ページ参照）を使うと，プレゼンテーションの展開がわかりやすくなります．（Unit 2〜Unit 5 でさらに詳しく説明します）

ポイント 適切な定型フレーズの使用は，聴き手の興味，関心を促し内容理解を深めるのに効果的です．

Tips プレゼンテーションの冒頭と終わりでは，挨拶だけでなくスマイルも忘れずに！

 先輩からのアドバイス

発表時間は守りましょう．話しすぎて時間超過するのは，座長，学会，あとの演者，何より聴衆に迷惑をかけることになります．

Presentation tips : Useful phrases

There are many useful phrases to structure the entire presentation.

Take a look at some examples for useful phrases for presentations.

Useful phrases for presentations

Opening Phrase	
Welcoming/Greeting	• Hello. Welcome to my presentation. • Hi, thank you all for coming to my presentation.
Introducing yourself	• Let me introduce myself. I'm a graduate student at ...
Presentation topic	• This presentation is about ... • Today, I'd like to talk about ...
Timing	• This presentation will take about 20 minutes.
Goals and outcomes	• By the end of this presentation, you will find ... • This presentation is relevant to those of you ...
Question	• If you have any questions, feel free to ask me at any time. • There will be a time for questions at the end of the presentation.
Outline/Structure	• As you see, this presentation has four sections.
Closing Remarks	• This is the end of my presentation. Thank you very much for your time and attention.

Transition phrases for presentations

Beginning	• First of all, I'll begin by...
In the middle	• Next ... • And then, • Let's move on to the next section.
Ending	• Finally, • I'll end with ... • In conclusion,

プレゼンテーションのはじめや終わりの部分で使える便利な定型フレーズを見てみましょう.

英語プレゼンテーションに役立つ定型フレーズ

はじめの挨拶,聴き手への感謝を伝える	• Hi/Hello. Welcome to my presentation. (訳) こんにちは. 私のプレゼンテーションにようこそお越しくださいました. • Hi/Hello. Thank you all for coming to my presentation. (訳) こんにちは. 本日はお越しいただきありがとうございます.
自己紹介	• Let me introduce myself. My name is [Fist Name], [Last Name]. I am a graduate student at [Name of your school]. (訳) 自己紹介をさせていただきます. 私は, [　　　] と申します. [　　　] の大学院生です.
プレゼンテーションのトピックについて聴き手に説明する	• This presentation is about [　　　]. (訳) このプレゼンテーションは, [　　　] についてです. • Today, I'd like to talk about [　　　]. I'm going to be talking about [　　　]. (訳) 本日, 私は [　　　] についてお話します.
所要時間	• This presentation will take about [　] minutes. (訳) このプレゼンテーションは [　] 分程度です. • I'll try to keep it short. (訳) 短めにお話します.
聴き手を引き込む,聴き手の興味や関心を高める	• By the end of this presentation, you will find [　　　]. (訳) このプレゼンテーションの終わりには, [　　　] がおわかりいただけるでしょう. • This presentation is relevant to those of you who [　　　]. (訳) このプレゼンテーションは, [　　　] をされている方々に関連した内容です.
質疑応答の仕方の説明	• There will be a time for questions at the end of the presentation. (訳) このプレゼンテーションの最後に質疑応答の時間があります.
アウトライン	• As you see, this presentation has four sections. (訳) ご覧のとおり, このプレゼンテーションには 4 つのセクションがあります.
終わりの挨拶	• This is the end of my presentation. Thank you for your attention. (訳) これでプレゼンテーションは終わりです. ご静聴ありがとうございました.

英語プレゼンテーションに使われるつなぎのフレーズ

はじめに	• First of all, I'll begin by [　　　]. (訳) まず, 私は [　　　] についての話をします.
次 に	• Next ...　(訳) 次の ... • And then,　(訳) それから, • Let's move on the next section.　(訳) 次のセクションにいきましょう
終わりに	• Finally,　(訳) 最後に, • I'll end with [　　　]. (訳) 私は [　　　] の話で終わります. • In conclusion,　(訳) 結論は,

B Body language: Gestures and eye contact
How do you use body language effectively in your presentation?

 効果的な話し方や態度について英語で読んでみましょう.

Even though you may have great presentation tools, you still need to work on how to speak to your audience. Expressions, such as body language and eye contact are also a kind of communication tool. A good presentation is not all about slides and technical skills. As we discussed earlier, a good and meaningful presentation could affect the audience's life, decision making, problem solving and their future. When giving your presentation, it's important to connect with your audiences and see their reactions. Another presentation method to approach to your audience is "expressions." Using expressions effectively will likely increase the opportunity that the audience becomes more engaged and interested in your presentation.

Let's try practicing expressions without the use of words!

Body language:
- Hand gestures (pointing index fingers, thumbs up sign, steepling)
- Facial expression (smile, noddig)
- Confident posture (stance)
- Arm placement
- Silence, purposeful pauses

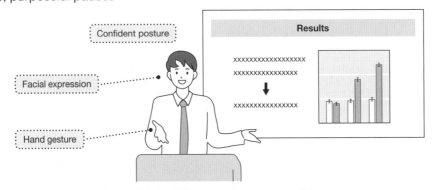

Appropriate body language shows your confidence.

Eye contact with your audience:
Make eye contact with the audience from right to left and left to right.

Tone of voice and speed:
- Resonant voice
- Volume (not too soft or loud)
- Adequate speed

話すことがらを整理してプレゼンテーションの構成ができたら，次は話し方についてですね．人前で話すの苦手だし，緊張するんですけど…

 最初に説明したように，プレゼンテーションは聴き手の行動変容を促すものです．原稿（script）をただ読んでいるだけでは，プレゼンテーションの対象の反応を確認しながら話すことができません．聴き手を見ながら話すようにしましょう．これをアイコンタクト（eye contact）とよびます．

アイコンタクト！気をつけます．たとえば，言葉だけで表現することが難しいとき，ボディーランゲージ（body language）を使っても構いませんか？

 もちろん．プレゼンテーションでは，ボディーランゲージを使うことで，聴き手に重要なポイントを伝えやすくなったり，関心をもたせる効果があります．

わかりました．ほかにも何か効果的に話す手法がありますか？

 声のトーンや話すスピードを変えるなどすることも効果的です．それから，聴き手が見やすい位置に立って正しい姿勢（posture）で話すことも大事です．せっかく視覚的効果の高いスライドを作成しても，聴き手にスライドが見えないと困りますね．

つまり，プレゼンテーションのスライドや原稿に依存するだけでは，聴き手の印象に残る，わかりやすいプレゼンテーションはできないってことですね！ちょっと恥ずかしいけど，声を出して練習したいと思います．

 次のセクションでは，もっと専門的な練習方法を紹介しますね．

ポイント ボディーランゲージやアイコンタクトなどの身ぶり，手ぶり，表情は，会話だけでなく，プレゼンテーションにおいても，聴き手にプレゼンの内容や重要なポイントを伝える効果的なテクニックです．以下のようなボディーランゲージを使って，表現（expressions）の練習をしてみましょう．鏡を見ながら練習するとより効果的です．

- ハンドジェスチャー（手を使う）
  例：大きさや長さを表現・いいね！を表現
- フェイシャルエクスプレッション（顔の表情を使う）
  例：眉毛や口角の上下運動し，喜怒哀楽を表現
- ポスチャー（姿勢・立ち方）
  例：背筋をまっすぐに正し，自信のある様子を表現
- アーム プレイスメント（腕の動きを使う）
  例：左右対称に手を合わせて，落ち着いている様子を表現
- ポーズ（間）
  例：トピックが変わるときに間をとる
- アイコンタクト（視線）
  例：会場全体を左右に見渡し，聴き手とコミュニケーションをとる表現
- 声の調子と話すスピード
  例：通る声，適度な速さ

注意点：
- 身ぶり・手ぶりは，大きく，ゆっくり，ほどほどに使う
- どの話をしているときに使うかをあらかじめ決めておく
- 文化によってジェスチャーの意味が異なるので，国際的な会合では特に気をつける

あまり使いすぎると，時間をかけて作成したプレゼンテーションのスライドや話の内容に聴き手が集中できなくなってしまいます．スピーキングをサポートする程度に使用するテクニックを身につけましょう．

Prosody

What speaking technique facilitates the listening comprehension and understanding of your audience?

 効果的な話し方をさらに掘り下げて，プロソディ（prosody）について読んでみましょう.

When you listen to a song, you can enjoy the sounds, rhythms, words, etc. The song has multiple elements, but the listener can understand the whole tune without any confusion. Do you know why? It's because of "prosody." The prosody in speaking is linguistically defined as rhythm and intonation. Considering how to speak to audiences is very important to your presentation. Three key points are: ❶ Pause, ❷ Stress, and ❸ Emphasis.

❶ **Pause** — Insert a *pause* after each chunk.
- Sentences that cannot be pronounced in one breath are divided into meaningful chunks.
- One chunk is pronounced in one breath. (e.g., Life science is / a branch of science...)

❷ **Stress** — Add a *stress* to create a natural rhythm.
- Establish a rhythm by pronouncing content words strongly and function words moderately.
- Content words and function words can be classified by parts of speech in principle.

Content and function words

Content words	Function words
- Noun	- Article
- Verb	- Preposition
- Adjective	- Auxiliary verb
- Adverb	- Pronoun
- 5W1H (Who, When, Where, What, Why, How)	- Relative pronoun
- Negatives (e.g., no, not, never)	- Copulative conjunction (e.g., and, so)

❸ **Emphasis** — Put an *emphasis* on key elements.
- Emphasize important words in a sentence. A word can be emphasized by raising your voice or taking a breath right before it. You can also speed up or slow down to emphasize a word.

話し方（スピーキング）は，話し手と聴き手の双方向の
コミュニケーションに影響します．少し専門的になりま
すが，初対面の相手にも聞き取りやすい話し方を練習す
るのにとてもいい方法，プロソディ（prosody）について
紹介をしましょう！

プロソディ？ 聞いたこともないですが，ぜひ教えてくだ
さい！ 実は，原稿をひたすら棒読みしてしまうくせが
あって困ってるんです．いい練習方法や話し方について
もっと知りたかったんです．

では，さっそくプロソディについて一緒に学びましょう．
プロソディとは，韻律のことです．

プロソディには重要な点が3つあります．
1つ目は chunk（意味のかたまり）ごとに区切りを入れ
る（**pause**）．
2つ目は **stress**（強勢）を置くことによって英語らしい
リズムをつける．
3つ目は大事なポイント **emphasis**（強調）を置く．

そっか！ 今まで一つひとつの単語を発音するのに必死
で，区切りについて考えていませんでした．たしかに日
本語でも，区切り方って大事ですね．「むかしむ / かしあ
るとこ / ろにおじいさんとお / ばあさんが住ん / でいま
した．」だと聞いているほうは意味が取れませんね．

そうです．たとえば，英語で話すときは，こんな感じに
なりますね．
Life science is / a branch of science // that deals with
living organisms.
大きな区切りは // ですが，"Life science" も長い語句で
しかも主語なので，一息で言いましょう．

❶ Pause（区切り）
- 一息に発音できない文は，意味区
  切りでフレーズに区切る
- 一つのフレーズは一気に発音す
  る．区切るのはフレーズとフレー
  ズの間のみ．

❷ Stress（強勢）
内容語を強く発音し，機能語は弱く
発音することによってリズムを確立
する．おもに内容を示す語とおもに
機能を示す語は，原則的に品詞で分
類できる．

内容を示す	機能を示す
・名 詞	・冠 詞
・動 詞	・前置詞
・形容詞	・助動詞
・副 詞	・代名詞
・疑問詞(5W1H)	・関係代名詞
・否定語(no, not, never, etc.)	・つなぎ言葉 (and, so, etc.)

❸ Emphasis（強調）
文の中で重要な単語を強調する（声
を高めたり，その前で一呼吸置くと
強調できる）．

D Prosody: Practice (Introductory level)

 Prosody の 3 原則を一つずつ練習しましょう.

Practice 1 Let's practice speaking. Read the following example, paying attention to the chunks.

Example: "Life science is a branch of science that deals with living organisms."

Pause (/)

> Life science is / a branch of science // that deals with living organisms.
> (/ pause, // longer pause)

"Life science" is a long phrase and the subject of the sentence, so it can be combined into one chunk.

Practice 2 Now, add *stress* to the example.

Chunk + Stress ( )

> Correct: Life science is / a branch of science // that deals with living organisms.
> Incorrect: Li fe sci en ce i s / a b ran ch of ......

Practice 3 The final step is to add *emphasis*.

Chunk + Stress + Emphasis (_)

In order to add emphasis, pronouncing only the accented syllable strongly.

Emphasize important words in a sentence (e.g., fields of study)

> Life science is / a branch of science // that deals with living organisms.

Please review more about prosody in Unit 3.

前項にひきつづき，プロソディのポイントを見ていきましょう．今度は stress を加えてみてください．

じゃあ，ハイライトしてみます．こんな感じですか？
Life science is / a branch of science // that deals with living organisms.

そうそう．ただ，life science と living organisms のように意味的に切り離すことが難しいフレーズは，一つの語のように続けて読むようにしましょう．
ちょっと発音してみましょうか？

はい！ ラ・イ・フ・サ・イ・エ・ン・ス / イズ ァ ブ・ラ・ン・チ オヴ …

あー，ちょっ，ちょっと待って！ stress をかける語は，そのすべての音節を大きな声で発音するのではなく，アクセント部分だけを強く発音しましょう．

すみません！道理で，なんか疲れるなって思いました …
Life science is / a branch of science // that deals with living organisms.
なんか，それっぽくなってきたでしょうか？

とてもいい感じになりましたね！次に emphasis を加えてみましょう！どの単語に emphasis をつけるかは，たとえ同じ文でも時と場合，相手によって変わります．今回は生命科学が特に生き物（living organisms）を扱う学問だということを伝えたいと思います．

Life science / is a branch of science // that deals with living organisms. これでどうでしょう？

Good Job！ Unit 3 でさらに練習していきましょう．

ポイント プロソディの 3 原則を理解し，さらに英語らしく話せるようになりましょう！

Tips プロソディの練習
● プレゼンテーションに役立つフレーズの例（p.21）やプロソディの例文を使って，どこに "内容語" と "機能語" があるかを分析してみましょう．
● 自分の研究分野で使用される専門的な用語で，特に英語で発音がしにくい単語のアクセントの部分を辞書で調べておきましょう．
● プレゼンテーションの原稿を読むとき，文のどこに "区切り" をいれると聴き手が聴きやすいか，読んで確認しましょう．
● 区切りのなかでも "どの言葉を強調するか" を決めて読んでみましょう．主張したいことや重要なポイントが聴き手に伝わるか，"強調する部分" を読んで確認しましょう．

Tips 日本語には，「橋」と「箸」と「端」のように，ピッチとよばれる音の高低のアクセントの違いで意味が変わる言葉があります．英単語は，音の高低に stress（強勢）が加わって意味が変わったり，品詞が変わったりします．プレゼンテーションの "present" という単語を例に，辞書で調べてみましょう．
● 名詞・形容詞の present
　［音節］pres·ent
　［発音とアクセント］préznt
● 動詞の present
　［音節］pri·ˈzent
　［発音とアクセント］prizént

1・5 実　践
自己紹介の練習をする

Practice

 下記のガイダンスに沿って自己紹介の練習をしましょう．
（難しい場合は先に右ページを読んでください）

Task 1・1 "Who you are?" 1-minute self-introduction

Tips: Keep it simple, keep it short, speak out, show your energy, do not read your script, do not forget eye contact and use body language.

Step 1 Fill-in the blanks and create your self-introduction script.

Step 2 Practice with your friends and classmates.

Step 3 Give feedback and comments to each other. What part of your self-introduction was good or needs to be improved?

Hi, I'm (First Name, Last Name). I am a (school year) studying (major) at (university/school name) in (city and country). I am a member of a/the (name of lab). My research interests focus on (fields of study). In particular, I'm interested in (specific subject, research topic and goal). My current research explores (current research topic). Besides my studies, I participate in a/the (students club name) club activity to (what you would like to share. what you would like to achieve). After graduating from university, I plan to (future plan/future career goal). Nice to meet you!

実際に練習してみましょう.

タスク 1・1　**1分くらいで，簡単な自己紹介をしてみましょう**

注意事項：発表時間，印象，聴き手への配慮，原稿をひたすら読まない，聴き手に好感をもたれる姿勢や態度，聴き手にわかりやすい話し方（プロソディ），アイコンタクトやボディーランゲージを使う

練習方法：

Step 1 （　）のところを英語にして，自己紹介のスクリプトをつくってみましょう

Step 2 プロソディに気をつけて，おたがいに自己紹介の練習をしてみましょう

Step 3 良かった点，改善したほうがいい点，そのほか入れたほうがいいことなどについて，おたがいにフィードバックやコメントをしましょう

Hi, I'm (名前，名字). I am a (学年) studying (専攻) at (大学名) in (大学の所在地).
I am a member of a/the (研究室名). My research interests focus on (おもに興味のある研究分野名). In particular, I'm interested in (そのなかでも特に興味のある研究トピックなど). My current research explores (現在の研究トピック名). Besides my studies, I participate in a/the (部活やサークル名) club activity to achieve (将来の目標など). After graduating from university, I plan to (卒業後にしたいことや卒業後の計画). Nice to meet you!

- -

例　Hi, I am Hana Hirayama. I am a senior* studying life sciences at Horinouchi University in Tokyo, Japan. I am a member of the biotechnology laboratory. My research interests focus on bioenergy science. In particular, I'm interested in the role of microbiology in achieving the UN SDGs (United Nations Sustainable Development Goals). My current research explores botanical power generation for environmental sustainability. Besides my studies, I participate in the entrepreneurship club to achieve my future goal of starting a business. After graduating from university, I plan to go to graduate school. Nice to meet you.

和訳　みなさん，こんにちは．堀ノ内大学生命科学部4年の平山ハナと申します．バイオテクノロジー研究室に所属しております．おもな研究分野は生命エネルギー分野です．特に，国連SDGs（持続可能な開発目標）の達成におけるマイクロバイオロジーの役割について興味があります．私は現在，環境の持続可能性のための植物発電について研究しています．研究以外では，学内の大学のアントレプレナーサークルに所属し，将来起業することを目標に活動をしております．卒業後は大学院に進学したいと考えております．どうぞよろしくお願いいたします．

＊英語で大学の1年生から4年生を以下のように表現します．
　1年生 freshman，2年生 sophomore，3年生 junior，4年生 senior

 学会などで研究の発表をするときの自己紹介については，Unit 2 で詳しく説明します.

Oral presentation
－Opening
プレゼンターとスタディの紹介

2・1 目　　的
プレゼンテーションの始め方を知る

A　Setting the stage of your presentation

Unit 2 から Unit 5 では，口頭発表（oral presentation）を下図に示す 4 セクションに分けて，各セクションで用意するスライドや話す内容について学んでいきます．Unit 2 では，まず Opening セクションをマスターしましょう．
右ページにある ▶◀ video 1 のプレゼンテーションをサンプルとして解説していきますので，video 1 を見てから始めましょう．

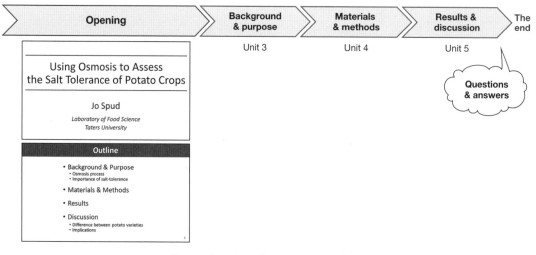

Preparation stages for your presentation

Functions

The opening section introduces the presenter / presentation.

In order to grab the attention of your audience:

1. Introduce the presenter effectively.
2. Provide an overview of the presentation.

オープニング（Opening）セクションの目的って何ですか？

 自分のプレゼンテーションの舞台をセットアップすることです．これを達成すると，聴き手は最後まで発表者のプレゼンテーションに集中することができます．特に，たがいに面識のない状況でのプレゼンテーションでは，Opening セクションで聴き手に適切な印象を与え，興味をひきつけることは必須ですね．

プレゼンテーションでも「最初が肝心」なんですね．でも，具体的には，どんなことをすれば自分の舞台のセットアップができるのでしょうか？

 ポイントは 2 つあります．プレゼンテーションは，発表者の紹介から始まります．他者から紹介される場合でも自己紹介する場合でも，自分が最初に話す際に重要なのは，「聴き手の心を掴む」ということです．そのために具体的にはどのように話すといいと思いますか？

たとえば，自己紹介をするときにちょっと面白いことを言って，聴いている人の笑いを誘うようにするとかですか？

 それもストラテジーの一つだと思いますが，一般的には，「聴き手の心を掴む」ために話すことは，自分の発表内容と関連のあることにします．そして，自分がこれから発表するトピックに関しては，エキスパートである，ということを印象づけることが重要です．

2 つ目のポイントは何ですか？

 プレゼンテーションの概要を伝える，ということです．どのような順番で発表を進めていくかを伝えることにより，観客は「聴く準備」ができます．プレゼンテーションの道筋を示すということです．限られた時間の中で十分に自分の主張を伝えるためには，発表を論理的に組み立てる必要があり，それを観客と共有しておくことで，わかりやすいプレゼンテーションにすることができます．

見てみよう

プレゼンテーションを 2 つ見てみましょう．
❶ Presentation 1：Osmosis
「ジャガイモの浸透圧を測ることにより塩耐性を調べた」という研究．このプレゼンをサンプルとして Unit 2 〜 Unit 5 を学んでいきます．

 video 1
Presentation 1
Osmosis

❷ Presentation 2：Phagocytosis
「ある酵素がマクロファージの貪食作用を制御している」という研究．

 video 2
Presentation 2
Phagocytosis

学習ガイド Unit 2 〜 Unit 5 は，以下のような構成になっています．
Unit 2：オープニング（Opening）
Unit 3：背景と目的（Background & purpose）
Unit 4：実験材料と方法（Materials & methods）
Unit 5：結果と考察（Results & discussion）

Unit 2 では，Title スライドと Outline スライドの 2 種類とそれぞれの作り方，話す内容，使用する表現を学習します．

ポイント オープニング（Opening）セクションの目的
• 聴き手の心を掴む
1）プレゼンターを紹介する
2）プレゼンテーションの概要を伝える

A　**Title slide**：Title, presenter's name, affiliation, etc.

 ここでは，スライドのサンプルを見ながらスライドに書くことを学びます．
まず Title スライドに書くべき情報を確認しましょう．

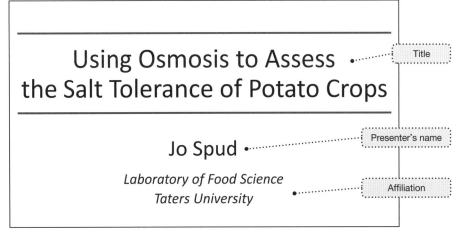

Title slide

Format

1）**Title**
 - Sentence form
 - Phrase form

2）**Capitalization**
 - Sentence case："Using osmosis to access the salt tolerance of potato crops"
 - Title case：　　"Using Osmosis to Access the Salt Tolerance of Potato Crops"

3）**Fonts**
 - San-serif（Arial, Helvetica）

タイトル（Title）スライドには何を書きますか？

 左ページのサンプルを見ながら確認してみましょう．情報が3つ載せてありますね．まず，プレゼンテーションのタイトル，そして，発表者の名前，最後が発表者の所属機関の名称です．

このほかに，プレゼンテーションを行う日の日付や場所を書くこともあります．また，学会やセミナーなどで発表する場合には，それらの情報を載せることもあります．自分の所属，大学，学会などの名称は正しく表記することが重要です．

プレゼンテーションのタイトルが大きく示されています．これはこのスライドで一番重要ということですか？

 そうですね．Opening セクションの目的を思い出してください．

観客の心を掴むために，自分のプレゼンテーションが何に関することかを視覚的に印象付けることは重要です．タイトルは，このスライドで最初に目に入る情報でしょう．そうなると，タイトルの付け方にも気を付ける必要があります．

タイトルの付け方の注意点とはどんなことですか？

 タイトルの付け方には次の2種類があります．「一文」で表すものと，「フレーズ」で示すものです．また，その表記の仕方，つまり大文字の使い方のルールもあります．タイトルの最初の文字のみ大文字にすることをセンテンスケース（sentence case）とよび，単語の最初の文字をそれぞれ大文字にすることをタイトルケース（title case）とよびます．

左のスライドの場合は，どんな付け方をしているでしょう？

タイトルは「フレーズ」で付けてあり，表記は単語の最初の文字がそれぞれ大文字になっているタイトルケースです．

 そうですね．語数，文字数制限など発表に当たってのルールを確認しておくことも忘れてはいけません．会場の大きさやスクリーンのサイズなど，できるだけ事前に確認して，フォントのサイズを検討することも大切ですね．

ポイント **Title** スライド

- プレゼンテーションタイトル
- 発表者の名前，所属
- 発表日時，場所
- 学会・セミナーなどの名称やその他情報
- 大学・所属機関や学会のロゴ

ポイント タイトルのフォーマット

1）タイトルの付け方
- 一文（sentence）

例：Enzyme X negatively regulates Fcγ receptor-mediated phagocytosis of murine macrophages

注意：ピリオドはつけない
- フレーズ（phrase）

例：Molecular characterization of protein Y in BRAF inhibitor-treated melanoma cells

2）大文字のルール
- センテンスケース

Using osmosis to access the salt tolerance of potato crops
- タイトルケース

Using Osmosis to Access the Salt Tolerance of Potato Crops

3）フォントの種類とサイズ
- 種類：装飾のない字体
- サイズ：大きいほうがいい

B Slide (1)：Outline

 Outline スライドに書くべき情報を確認しましょう.

Outline

- Background & Purpose
  - Osmosis process
  - Importance of salt-tolerance
- Materials & Methods
- Results
- Discussion
  - Difference between potato varieties
  - Implications

1

Slide（1）： Outline
(Optional depending on the type of presentation)

Functions

- Prepare the audience for your presentation.
1. Tell the audience the topic of your presentation.
2. Tell the audience the order in which your talk will follow.

アウトライン（Outline）スライドの目的は何ですか？

 聴き手に事前にプレゼンテーションでどのようなことがどのような順番で語られるかをあらかじめ伝えることです.

Outline スライドは必ず必要ですか？

 そんなことはないですよ.
短いプレゼンテーションの場合, Title スライドを見せながらプレゼンテーションの流れを説明することはよくあります. 時間が十分に与えられている場合は, Outline スライドがあったほうがわかりやすいです.

Outline スライドには何を書きますか？

 サンプル（左ページ）を見ながら確認してみましょう.
目次のようになっていますね.
"Background & purpose" には, 重要なポイントが 2 つ示されています. そして結果を考察する "Discussion" にも, 2 つのポイントがあります. これにより, 聴き手の「聴く準備」を整えることができますね.

ただ, Background & purpose, Materials & methods... のようにセクションだけを列挙するならば, Outline スライドを作成する意味がありません. 聴き手が聴く準備ができるように, ポイントを記載することが重要です.
スライドの書き方で, 何か気付いたことはありますか？

情報が列挙されているだけで, 文は書いてありません.

 そうですね. Outline スライドだけでなく, 基本的にスライドは箇条書きです. 完全文（full sentence）で書きません.

ポイント Outline スライド
参加者に自分のプレゼンテーションを聴く準備をさせる
• プレゼンテーションの内容を簡潔に伝える
　→ポイントだけ列挙する（文は使わない）
• プレゼンテーションで話す内容の順序を伝える

注意事項 Outline スライドをつくるときには…
• 発表時間を考えて使用の有無を判断する
• セクション（Background & purpose, Materials & methods …）だけを列挙することは避ける（内容のポイントを入れる）

 先輩からのアドバイス

プレゼンテーションのどのセクションにおいても, スライドの目的は, 話す内容を簡潔に示し, 話していることがより明確に伝わるようにすることです. スライドに「文」を並べてしまうと, 聴き手はスライドを"読む" ことに気を取られてしまい, 発表者の話を聞くことに集中できません. もっと悪いことに, 発表者自身がスライドを読んでしまうことにもなりかねません. スライドは, 情報を視覚的に示すものであり, 原稿ではないことに留意しましょう.

2・3 話す準備
話すことがらを知る

Preparation of script

> 話すことがらを準備するために，まず標準的な話の展開を知りましょう．右ページを読んでから，下の Move pattern を確認していきましょう．

A Move analysis：Title slide

Move pattern

- Move 1：Starter
    - Step 1：Greetings
    - Step 2：Welcome remarks
- Move 2：Self introduction
    - Step 1：Presenter's name
    - Step 2：Affiliation
    - Step 3：Area of research
- Move 3：Introduction of the presentation
    - Step 1：Presentation topic
    - Step 2：Significance of the research

Variation

- Move 1：Starter
    - Step 1：Addressing gratitude for introduction
    - Step 2：Greetings
- Move 2：Significance of the research

これから話す準備をしましょう．ここでは Move を使って説明していきます．

Move ってなんですか？

話の展開の単位を Move といいます．Move をさらに細かく Step に分けることもあります．左のページに Title スライドの一般的な Move 構成（Move pattern）を示しています．Title スライドはプレゼンテーションのタイトルと発表者の紹介でしたね．

Move 1：Starter から見ましょう．ここには Step が 2 つあります．
参加者に向けて，まず最初に言うことはなんでしょうか？

とりあえず，Hello っていいます．

それが Step 1：Greetings「挨拶」です．
つづいて，Step 2：Welcome remarks「来場に対する感謝の一言」です．プレゼンテーションを聞きに来てくれた参加者に向けて "Thank you for coming to my presentation." と，謝意を伝えます．これらをまとめて Move 1：Starter とよびます．
Move 2：Self introduction は名前，所属，自分の研究分野を伝えます．
Move 3：Introduction of the presentation はプレゼンテーションのトピックの紹介です．ここで，プレゼンテーションのタイトルを伝えることもあります．

Move とそれを細分化した Step を見るとどんな項目をどんな順序で伝えるかがわかりますね．

そうです．Unit 2 から Unit 5 ではプレゼンテーションを構成する Move と Step を紹介します．いつ何をどの順番で伝えればよいかがわかるようになります．

実際のプレゼンテーションでは司会者が発表者を紹介することも多いので，その際の Move も見ておきましょう．左ページ "Variation" の Move では，司会者がプレゼンテーションの前に，発表者の名前，所属，研究分野を紹介していることが前提です．その場合，Move 1 の Starter は「司会者に対する謝辞」になります．そして，Move 2 のプレゼンテーション内容の紹介へつなげます．

ポイント **Move とは**
- 話の展開の単位
- Move はさらに細かく Step に分けることもある

Move pattern Title スライド
- Move 1：開 始
  - Step 1：挨 拶
  - Step 2：来場に対する感謝の一言
- Move 2：自己紹介
  - Step 1：発表者の名前
  - Step 2：所 属
  - Step 3：研究分野
- Move 3：発表の紹介
  - Step 1：発表トピック
  - Step 2：本研究の意義

バリエーション
- Move 1：開 始
  - Step 1：司会者への謝辞
  - Step 2：挨 拶
- Move 2：本研究の意義

B Script: Title slide

Title スライドの Move 構成をさらに掘り下げます．右ページを読んで，
タスクに挑戦しましょう．

Task 2·1 **Move analysis**: Title slide

Divide the script into moves and steps. The first move has been indicated for you. Then, check the items you used in the "Move pattern" below.

> _{Move 1 Step 1}   _{Move 1 Step 2}
> Good morning everyone, / and thank you for attending my presentation today. / My name is Jo Spud, / and I work at the Laboratory of Food Science at Taters University. My main area of research is food chemistry. Today, I would like to show you how our team can use potatoes to illustrate the important process of osmosis and determine the salt concentration inside different types of potatoes. Our experiment can provide information on which potato crop is best to grow in high salt areas.

Move pattern

- ☑ Move 1: Starter
  - ☑ Step 1: Greetings
  - ☑ Step 2: Welcome remarks
- ☐ Move 2: Self introduction
  - ☐ Step 1: Presenter's name
  - ☐ Step 2: Affiliation
  - ☐ Step 3: Area of research
- ☐ Move 3: Introduction of the presentation
  - ☐ Step 1: Presentation topic
  - ☐ Step 2: Significance of the research

左ページに示したのは，§2・2Ａの Title スライド（p.34）に対応するスクリプトです．

このスクリプトを Move に分けてみましょう．

タスク 2・1

Move analysis：Title スライド

Move pattern を参考にして，左のスクリプトを Move と Step に分けましょう．使用した Move/Step にチェックマークを入れましょう．p.143 に模範解答があります．

Move 1：Starter を一緒にやっていきましょう．左ページの "Move pattern" を見てみましょう．この Move には Step が２つあります．スクリプトを見て，最初からどこまでが，Greetings に相当し，その次に Welcome remarks はどこまでかを考えてみましょう．

Greetings は「挨拶」ですから，挨拶の終わりに，/（スラッシュ）を入れます．これで区切りを示しましょう．そして，そこに "Move 1 Step 1" と書き込んでおきましょう．ここまでがひとつの「話の展開」になるわけです．その次は Welcome remarks ですね．来場に関する感謝を述べるわけですが，それの終わりに，スラッシュを入れます．ここも「話の展開」の区切りになります．先ほどと同じように，Move 1 Step 2 と書き込みましょう．

次は Move 2 で示してある Self introduction「自己紹介」，へと展開します．Move 1 と同じようにして，区切りを示して，どの Move/Step に相当するか書き込んでください．

C Move analysis: Slide (1) "Outline"

 つづいて Outline スライドの Move 構成を見ていきましょう.

Move pattern

- Move 1: Transition (Title → Outline)
- Move 2: Outline
    Step 1: Transition + Content 1
    Step 2: Transition + Content 2
    Step 3: Transition + Content 3
        ⋮
- Move 3: Significance of the research

Outline スライドの一般的な Move を紹介します（左ページ）．実験や調査の結果に基づいて発表する場合はこれをよく使います．
Move 1 では，Title スライドから次へ移ることを話します．この Move をトランジッション "Transition" とよびます．
Move 2 は Outline スライドでは何を話すかをステップに分けて示しています．

• Move 1：トランジッション
　　　　　　　　（Title → Outline）
• Move 2：アウトライン
　　Step 1：トランジッション＋内容 1
　　Step 2：トランジッション＋内容 2
　　Step 3：トランジッション＋内容 3
　　（ほかにも Step があれば追加する）
• Move 3：研究の重要性

トランジッションって具体的にはどんなことですか？

話の変わり目を示すものです．
次のスライドに進むとき，つまり，話題が転換するときに，どのように言えばいいでしょうか？

とりあえず，Next, I will talk about で始めます．

そうですね．ただし，同じ表現ばかり使うと，単調なプレゼンテーションになってしまいます．トランジッションにはさまざまな表現があるので，学習してどんどん増やしていきましょう．

"Content" とは何をさしていますか？

ここでの "Content" は，プレゼンテーションの内容のことです．ただ単に，話す順番を伝えるだけであれば，Outline スライドを作成する意味がないということは，すでに説明しましたね．聴き手の聞く準備が整うようにするのが Opening セクションの目的ですから，話す順番のなかでも特に重要なポイントを明確に伝えるようにします．それぞれのポイントが "Content" です．

D Script：Slide (1) "Outline"

Outline スライドの Move をさらに掘り下げます．右ページを読んで，タスクに挑戦しましょう．

Task 2·2 Move analysis：Slide (1)

Divide the script into moves and steps. The first move has been indicated for you. Then, check the items you used in the "Move pattern" below.

Move 1

I would like to begin by sharing with you the outline of my presentation. / I will first give you a brief overview of the process of osmosis, and explain why it's important to know the salt content of different potato varieties. Next, I will show how we used potatoes to demonstrate how osmosis works. Then, I will explain how this experiment allowed us to determine the unknown salt concentration of potatoes. These results could help to quickly check which crops are more tolerant of higher salt concentration, as well as to develop cheaper ways to measure salinity in other things.

Move pattern

- ☑ Move 1：Transition (Title → Outline)
- ☐ Move 2：Outline
    - ☐ Step 1：Transition + Content 1
    - ☐ Step 2：Transition + Content 2
    - ☐ Step 3：Transition + Content 3
- ☐ Move 3：Significance of the research

左ページに示したのは，§2・2 B の Slide (1)：Outline (p.36) に対応するスクリプトです．

このスクリプトを Move に分けてみましょう．

タスク 2・2

Move analysis：スライド(1)

Move pattern を参考にして，スクリプトを Move と Step に分けましょう．使用した Move/Step にチェックマークを入れましょう．p.143 に模範解答があります．

2・4 スピーキング
話し方のスキルを身につける

Speaking

A Voice quality and eye contact

 話す内容の次は話し方を学んでいきます．動画を見てタスクに挑戦しましょう．

Task 2・3 Video lesson

What did you notice?

 video 3
Task 2・3

Techniques

- Voice quality
  - Speak with a voice that reaches the audience.
  - Speak clearly.
- Eye contact
  - Use eye contact appropriately. Do not read the slides or scripts.

Task 2・4 Practice with the video

Watch the video and practice speaking paying attention to the skills
you learned in §1・4 and Task 2・3 above.

 video 4
Task 2・4

Task 2・5 Watch the video

Compare the two presentations. How are they different?

  video 5
Task 2・5

音声を聴いて，比べてみましょう.

| タスク 2・3 | **Video lesson** | ▶️ video 3 |

video 3 を見て，気づいたことをメモしましょう.

 Title スライドを提示しながら話す際のポイントとして，ここでは，以下に注意しましょう.

- 発 声
  聴き手に届く声を出す
  明瞭に話す
- アイコンタクト
  聴き手を見ながら話す
  スクリプト，スライドを読み上げない

| タスク 2・4 | **Practice with the video** | ▶️ video 4 |

上で学んだスキルを活用して，video 4 を見ながらモデルに合わせ何度も練習しましょう. 発音，プロソディ，話すスピードに気をつけましょう.

| タスク 2・5 | **Watch the video** | ▶️ video 5 |

video 5 を見て，2つのプレゼンテーションを比べましょう.

Opening セクションについて学んだことを実践しましょう.

Task 2・6 **Your presentation**

Work on the opening section of your own presentation. Use the following expressions. (See "Useful expressions" on p.146)

Title slide

■ Move 1: Starter	
Step 1: Greetings	‣ Good morning / Good afternoon everyone.
Step 2: Welcome remarks	‣ Thank you for attending my presentation today.
	‣ I'm very happy to have a chance to present my research on ...
■ Move 2: Self introduction	
Step 1: Presenter's name	‣ My name is ...　‣ I'm ...
Step 2: Affiliation	‣ I work at ...　　‣ I am a student / researcher at ...
Step 3: Area of research	‣ My main area of research is ...
■ Move 3: Introduction of the presentation	
Step 1: Presentation topic	‣ Today, I would like to share with you
Step 2: Significance of the research	‣ Our experiment / research / study can provide ...

Outline slide

■ Move 1: Transition (Title → Outline)	‣ Let me give you the outline of my presentation.
■ Move 2: Outline	
Step 1: Transition + Content 1	‣ First, (content 1)
Step 2: Transition + Content 2	‣ Next, (content 2)
Step 3: Transition + Content 3	‣ Then / Finally, (content 3)
■ Move 3: Significance of the research	‣ My/Our research could help ...

タスク 2・6	**Your presentation**

Opening セクションのスライドとスクリプトを作成しましょう．左ページに示した表現を使うことができます．必要に応じて，付録 A: 機能表現集（p.146）を参照しましょう．

(1) スライドのイメージ図を書いてみよう．

(2) スクリプトを書いてみよう．

Good afternoon everyone.

Thank you for _____ .

My name is _____

and I _____ .

My main area of research is _____ .

Today, I would like to share with you _____ .

Our （   ） can provide _____ .

I would like to begin by _____ .

I will first _____ .

Next, I will show _____ .

Then, I will explain _____ .

(And finally, I will summarize _____ .)

Our （   ） could help _____ .

Checklist

あなたが準備したスライド，スクリプト，そして話し方について，以下のことができているか確認しましょう．

☑ Slide design

☐	The title clearly describes what the presentation is about.	… タイトルが発表の内容を端的に示している
☐	Spelling and capitalization of the title are appropriate.	… タイトルが正確に書かれている（スペリング，大文字・小文字の使い方）
☐	The name (with title) of the presenter is correctly written.	… プレゼンターの名前（肩書き，称号含む）が書かれている
☐	The affiliation of the presenter is correctly written.	… 所属が正確に書かれている
☐	The outline shows the order in which the ideas are presented.	… 内容が話す順番に従って書かれている
☐	The content is written concisely.	… 内容が簡潔に書かれている
☐	The font type and size are appropriate.	… フォントの種類，サイズが適切である
☐	There are no unnecessary pictures or images on the slide.	… 不必要な絵を挿入していない

☑ Script

☐	The script contains appropriate moves and steps.	… 適切な Move/Step が使用されている
☐	The script follows the order of the slides.	… 話す順番がスライドの順番に沿っている
☐	The script sticks to the slide content.	… 話す内容がスライドと合っている

☑ Speaking

☐	Voice is loud and clear enough to reach the audience.	… 声がはっきりと十分に聴き手に届いている
☐	Eye contact is used appropriately.	… アイコンタクトを適切に使っている
☐	Presentation is given without reading slides or script.	… スライドやスクリプトを読まずに発表をしている

Unit 3

Oral presentation
―Background & purpose
背景と研究目的の紹介

3・1 目　的
今わかっていること，わかっていないことを明確にし，研究の目的を伝える

A Justifying the purpose of the research

3・2 スライドのデザイン
スライドに書くことを知る

A Slide (2)：Background (previous research and what we want to know)

B Slides (3), (4)：Key terms/concepts (definition/explanation of the key terms/concepts)

C Slide (5)：Objectives (research objectives, research questions or hypotheses)

3・3 話 す 準 備
話すことがらを知る

A Move analysis：Slide (2) to Slide (5)

B Script：Slide (2) "Background"

C Script：Slides (3), (4) "Key terms/concepts"

D Script：Slide (5) "Objectives"

3・4 スピーキング
話し方のスキルを身につける

A Prosody

3・5 実　践
練習をする

A　Justifying the purpose of the research

 Unit 3 では，Background & purpose セクションについて学んでいきます．
まずは目的をおさえましょう．

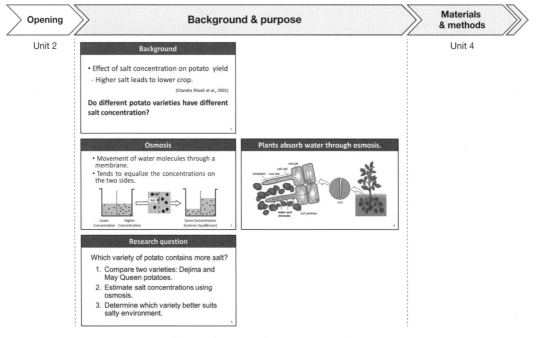

Preparation stages for your presentation

Functions

The background section introduces the background/purpose of the study.

- Clarify what we already know about the topic (previous research) and what we don't yet know.
- Explain the key terms and concepts used in the presentation.
- Indicate specific research objectives, research questions or hypotheses.

背景と目的（Background & purpose）セクションの目的って何ですか？

自分の研究を発表する土台をつくることです．具体的には，研究の必要性と研究目的を示します．

自分がなぜその研究テーマに興味をもったか，だけではダメなんですね．

そうです．まずは先行研究でどこまでわかっているかを述べたうえで，まだわかっていないこと示します．

なるほど，わかっていないことを示して，それを解明することが，これから発表する研究の目的だ，ということですね．

そのとおり．これまでにわかっていることから始めて，最後に具体的な研究目的を伝えます．
あと忘れてはいけないのが，研究に関わる基本概念・基本用語を説明することです．自分のプレゼンテーションを聴く人がどんな知識をもっているかを先に把握することが大切です．

ポイント 背景と目的（Background & purpose）セクションの目的

- テーマについてすでにわかっていること（先行研究）とまだわかっていないことを明確にする
- 発表で使うおもな用語や概念を解説する
- 具体的な研究目的（リサーチクエスチョンや仮説など）を示す

Background & purpose セクションではどんなスライドが必要でしょうか？
まず，このセクション全体の流れをつかみましょう．

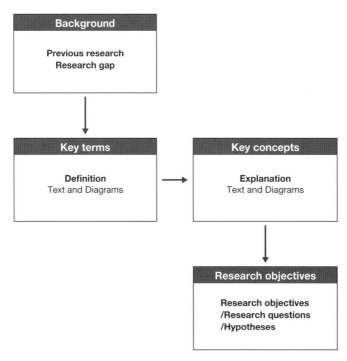

Information flow

Format

1) Background slide：Previous research；Research gap
2) Key terms/concepts slide：Explanation using text and diagrams
3) Research objectives slide：Research objectives/Research questions/Hypotheses

スライドがたくさんありますね．どのスライドに何を書けばいいですか？

 まず全体の流れを予習しましょう．
背景を示すスライドには，まず先行研究（previous research）に基づいてすでにわかっていることを示します．そしてわかっていないこと（リサーチギャップ research gap）を示し，次に基本用語や概念（key terms/concepts）のスライドで，背景知識を説明します．
最後に研究目的（research objectives）を示すスライドで具体的な研究目的を示します．

えーっと，リサーチギャップと研究目的の違いがわかりません．まだわかっていないことは研究目的にならないんですか？

 いい質問ですね．たとえばケーキの材料である砂糖が甘味のほかにケーキの出来にどう作用するかわかっていないとします．これがリサーチギャップです．これを解明するために，少し焦点を絞ってスポンジケーキをさまざまな分量の砂糖で焼き，焼き上がりの高さを比較した．つまり，具体的な研究目的は，スポンジケーキの高さに砂糖の分量がどんな影響を与えるかを調べることです．

なるほど，リサーチギャップから焦点を絞ったものが研究目的なんですね．

 そういうことです．スライド(2)（次ページ参照）ではリサーチギャップを先行研究と同じスライドに示していますが，発表内容に応じて変えられます．ただし研究目的を示す前でなければいけません．それでは，それぞれのスライドを詳しく見ていきましょう．

ポイント Background & purpose
セクションのスライド構成
• **Background** スライド：先行研究およびすでにわかっていること，まだわかっていないこと（リサーチギャップ）を示す
• **Key terms/concepts** スライド：基本用語，基本概念の解説を図や文で示す
• **Research objectives** スライド：研究目的，リサーチクエスチョン，仮説を示す

A **Slide (2)： Background** (previous research and what we want to know)

研究の背景を説明する Background スライドを見ていきましょう.

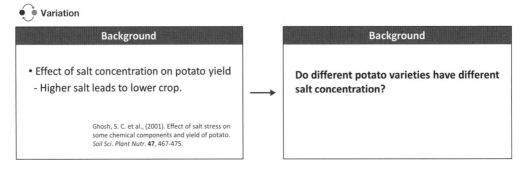

Background

• Effect of salt concentration on potato yield
 - Higher salt leads to lower crop.

(Chandra Ghosh et al., 2001)

Do different potato varieties have different salt concentration?

2

Slide（2）： Background

● ● Variation

Background
• Effect of salt concentration on potato yield 　- Higher salt leads to lower crop. Ghosh, S. C. et al., (2001). Effect of salt stress on some chemical components and yield of potato. *Soil Sci. Plant Nutr.* **47**, 467-475.

→

Background
Do different potato varieties have different salt concentration?

Another way to show previous research and research gap

Functions
• The background slides show what we know so far.
• Cite any previous research properly.
• Describe what we do not know (research gap).
• A research gap can be placed on the same slide with previous research.

ではまず背景を示すスライドから説明しますね. 左ページを見てください.
この例では，これまでにわかっていること（先行研究）とリサーチギャップを1枚のスライドにまとめました.

上がこれまでにわかっていることで，太字で示した文がまだわかっていないことですね. そして，場合によってはこれを2枚のスライドに分けてよいということですね.

そうですね. "Variation" に示したとおりです.

スライドの中ほどのカッコで示されているのは何ですか？

これは先行研究の出典です. これまでにわかっていることは，土壌の塩分濃度がジャガイモの生産量にどう影響するかを調べた結果，塩分濃度が高いほど生産量が低かったということですが，それが誰の研究結果か，その出典をカッコの中に示しています.
出典は，2001年に発表された Chandra Ghosh 氏とその他複数の研究者による研究ということです. "et al." は筆頭著者である Chandra Ghosh さんのほかに共著者が複数いることを示しています.

このスライドで，リサーチギャップは疑問文で示されていますが，疑問文と決まっているのですか？

"Salt concentration of different varieties of potatoes are not known." でもよいです.

ポイント **Background** スライド
〔スライド(2)〕
• これまでにわかっていることとわかっていないこと（リサーチギャップ）を示す. それぞれ別のスライドでも可.
• これまでにわかっていることは出典を明記すること.
• リサーチギャップは先行研究と同じスライドに記載する場合もある.
• 引用文献は著者名と出版年だけを示す場合と，論文タイトルやジャーナル名を含むすべての書誌情報を入れる場合がある.
• 引用文献の書き方は分野によって異なる.

Slides (3), (4) : Key terms/concepts
(definition / explanation of the key terms / concepts)

次は，研究を理解してもらうために必要な用語や基本概念を示す
Key terms/concepts スライドを見ていきましょう．

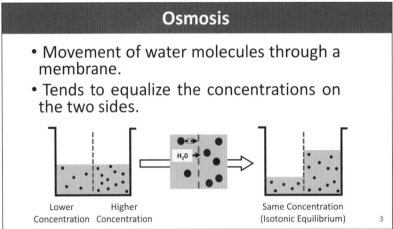

When defining the key term, put the term as the slide title.

Slide (3) : **Key terms /concepts**

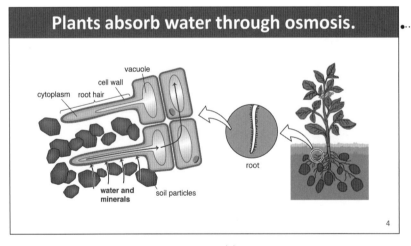

When explaining the key concept, put the concept as the slide title.

Slide (4) : **Key terms /concepts**

Functions

- Key terms/concepts slides explain important terms and concepts for your presentation.
- Decide which terms or concepts to explain considering what your audience may know.
- Diagrams are easier to understand.
- Key terms/concepts slides can be placed before or after the background slides.

次は基本用語・基本概念を説明するスライドです.
このプレゼンテーションでは,基本用語として osmosis（浸透作用）の意味と,基本概念として植物の中でosmosis によって何が起こっているかを示します.1枚目は osmosis の作用を図で表したもの,2枚目では植物の毛根が osmosis によって土壌の中の水や養分を吸い上げることを図示していますね.

図で示してあるのでわかりやすいですね.

聴き手の負担を軽くするために,文で説明するよりも目で見てわかる図を使うとよいです.

ちょっと待ってください.説明するといってもどの程度説明すればいいのかわかりません.自分と同じテーマで研究している人なら基本用語・基本概念は説明しなくてもわかっていると思いますが,別の研究分野の人に対しては詳しい説明が必要だと思います.

いいことに気づきましたね!聴き手がどんな知識をもっている人なのか,立ち止まって考えてみることは重要ですね.

自分のプレゼンテーションを聴き手に理解してもらうためには基本用語・基本概念の説明を相手に合わせてしっかりするということですね.

このサンプルでは背景を示すスライド（p.56）のあとに基本用語と基本概念を説明するスライドを置きますが,場合によっては背景を示すスライドよりも先にそれらを説明するほうがよい場合もあるでしょう.

たしかに先行研究やリサーチギャップも基本用語・基本概念がわからないと理解できない場合がありますね.

ポイント Key terms/concepts スライド〔スライド(3), (4)〕
- 基本用語・概念の説明を示す
- 聴き手に合わせてどの用語・概念を説明するか,どう説明するかを変える
- 文だけでなく図を使うと一目瞭然でわかりやすい
- 基本用語・概念の説明を示すスライドは,背景を示すスライドの前に置いても後に置いてもよい

C Slide (5)：Objectives
(research objectives, research questions or hypotheses)

Background & purpose セクションの最後のスライドで研究目的を紹介しましょう．

Research question

Which variety of potato contains more salt?

1. Compare two varieties: Dejima and May Queen potatoes.
2. Estimate salt concentrations using osmosis.
3. Determine which variety better suits salty environment.

5

Slide （5）： Objectives

 Variation 1

Research objective
To identify which variety of potato contains more salt. 1. Compare two varieties: Dejima and May Queen potatoes. 2. Estimate salt concentrations using osmosis. 3. Determine which variety better suits salty environment.

 Variation 2

Hypothesis
The amount of salt may differ between Dejima and May Queen. 1. Compare two varieties: Dejima and May Queen potatoes. 2. Estimate salt concentrations using osmosis. 3. Determine which variety better suits salty environment.

Other ways to show objectives

Functions

- The objectives slide shows research objectives.
- You may also outline the basic research methodology.
- There are three ways to indicate objectives：research questions, research objectives, and hypotheses.

いよいよ研究目的の紹介ですね.

 そうです. 聴いている人たちも準備万端, 期待が高まってきたところで, 研究目的を紹介して焦点をぎゅっと絞りましょう.
左ページは研究目的を示すスライドのサンプルです. 最初の疑問文がリサーチクエスチョン（Research question）です. そのあと, 基本的な研究方法を示すこともあります.

なるほど, 1 から 3 のステップが基本的な研究方法なんですね. このステップを達成すると本研究の目的である "Which variety of potato contains more salt?" に答えられるんですね.

 今回は研究目的をリサーチクエスチョンとして疑問文で示しましたが, 左ページの "Variation" に示したとおり, 目的（Objectives）や仮説（Hypotheses）として疑問文以外で提示することもできます.
例（目的）: To identify which variety of potato contains more salt.
例（仮説）: The amount of salt may differ between Dejima and May Queen.

ポイント **Objectives** スライド〔スライド(5)〕
• 研究目的を示す
• 研究目的に加えて手順のステップごとに目的を示してもよい
• Objectives の示し方は "Research questions", "Objectives", "Hypotheses" の 3 種類ある

3・3 話 す 準 備
話すことがらを知る

Preparation of script

A **Move analysis: Slide (2) to Slide (5)**

 次は，Background & purpose セクションで話すことがらを準備するために，まず Move 構成を確認していきましょう.

Move pattern

- Move 1: Transition (Outline → Background)
- Move 2: Building on previous research
    Step 1: Findings of previous research
    Step 2: Research gap
- Move 3: Explanation of key terms/concepts
- Move 4: Research objectives

Variation

- Move 1: Transition (Outline → Background)
- Move 2: Explanation of key terms/concepts
- Move 3: Building on previous research
    Step 1: Findings of previous research
    Step 2: Research gap
- Move 4: Research objectives

このセクションの一般的な Move 構成を紹介します.

まずトランジッションです. Move 2 の Step1 でこれまでにわかっていることを明確にし, Step2 でこの分野で不足している知見…つまりまだわかっていないことを指摘します. 次に Move 3 でこの研究を理解するのに必要な基本用語・基本概念の説明をし, Move 4 で具体的な研究目的を "Research question" や "Hypotheses", "Objectives" の形式で述べます.

Move が入れ替わってもいいんですよね.

 そうです. 先にも話したように, 最初に基本用語・基本概念を説明してから先行研究の紹介をしても構いません.

あれ? このプレゼンテーションの場合ではどのスライドがどの Move にあたるのかな?

 整理してみましょう.
Move 1, Move 2: スライド(2) "Background"
Move 3: スライド(3), (4) "Osmosis" と "Plants absorb water through osmosis."
Move 4: スライド(5) "Research question"

なるほど, Move 1 と Move 2 は 1 枚のスライドにまとめられる, Move 3 は説明が必要な用語や概念の数だけスライドがあるということですね.

 そうです. スクリプトの Move を確認していきましょう.

Move pattern
Background & purpose セクション

- Move 1: トランジッション
  (Outline→Background)
- Move 2: 先行研究に基づいてリサーチギャップを示す
  Step1: 先行研究でわかったこと
  Step2: リサーチギャップ(まだわからないこと)
- Move 3: 基本用語・基本概念の説明
- Move 4: 研究目的

バリエーション

- Move 1: トランジッション
  (Outline→Background)
- Move 2: 基本用語・基本概念の説明
- Move 3: 先行研究に基づいてリサーチギャップを示す
  Step1: 先行研究でわかったこと
  Step2: リサーチギャップ(まだわからないこと)
- Move 4: 研究目的

B Script: Slide (2) "Background"

ここからは，Background & purpose セクションのスクリプトを読みながら，前項で紹介した Move 構成を具体的に分析していきます．タスクに挑戦しましょう．

Task 3·1 Move analysis: Slide (2)

Divide the script into moves and steps. The first move has been indicated for you. Then, check the items you used in the "Move pattern" below.

Move 1

Now, we come to the main section of my presentation. I will first explain the purpose of our study. / Previous research has established that higher salt concentration in the soil leads to a decrease in potato crop production. Getting more information about the salt concentration inside potatoes could help choose which variety is better suited to higher salt environments, as we can assume that varieties with higher salt content could be more tolerant of soils containing more salt.

Move pattern

☑ Move 1: Transition (Outline → Background)
☐ Move 2: Building on previous research
　　☐ Step 1: Findings of previous research
　　☐ Step 2: Research gap
☐ Move 3: Explanation of key terms/concepts
☐ Move 4: Research objectives

左ページに示したのは, §3・2 A の Slide (2)：Background (p.56) に対応するスクリプトです.

このスクリプトを Move に分けてみましょう.

タスク 3・1 **Move analysis：スライド(2)**

Move pattern を参考にして, スクリプトを Move と Step に分けましょう. 使用した Move/Step にチェックマークを入れましょう. p.143 に模範解答があります.

C Script: Slides (3), (4) "Key terms/concepts"

前項にひきつづき，Background & purpose セクションのスクリプトを読んで，Move 構成を分析しましょう．

Task 3·2 Move analysis: Slides (3), (4)
Divide the script into moves and steps. Then, check the items you used in the "Move pattern" below.

Before I go over our experiment's methods in detail, I will give you a brief explanation of the process of osmosis. Osmosis is the spontaneous movement of water molecules through a membrane from an area of lower concentration to an area of higher concentration. During osmosis, water moves through the membrane, but other molecules do not. This results in changes in concentration on both sides of the membrane. As you can see on this diagram, the movement of water tends to equalize the concentrations on the two sides of the membrane. This is the moment of isotonic equilibrium.

Here is an image of a plant with roots absorbing water. You can see root cells absorbing water and minerals through osmosis. A potato is a tuber of potato plant and is similar to a root. For osmosis to occur, the salt concentration of a potato needs to be higher than the salt concentration of the soil. Potatoes with high salt concentration can survive in salty soil, and can be planted in areas near ocean.

Move pattern

☐ Move 1: Transition (Outline → Background)
☐ Move 2: Building on previous research
　　☐ Step 1: Findings of previous research
　　☐ Step 2: Research gap
☐ Move 3: Explanation of key terms/concepts
☐ Move 4: Research objectives

左ページに示したのは，§3・2 B の Slides (3), (4)：Key terms/concepts（p.58）に対応するスクリプトです．

このスクリプトを Move に分けてみましょう．

タスク 3・2　**Move analysis**：スライド **(3)**，**(4)**

Move pattern を参考にして，スクリプトを Move と Step に分けましょう．使用した Move/Step にチェックマークを入れましょう．p.143 に模範解答があります．

D　Script : Slide (5) "Objectives"

前項にひきつづき，Background & purpose セクションのスクリプトを読んで，Move 構成を分析しましょう．

Task 3·3　Move analysis : Slide (5)

Divide the script into moves and steps. Then, check the items you used in the "Move pattern" below.

Here is the research question. Which variety of potato contains more salt?

1. Compare two varieties : Dejima and May Queen potatoes.

2. Estimate salt concentrations using osmosis.

3. Determine which variety better suits salty environment.

Move pattern

☐ Move 1 : Transition (Outline → Background)
☐ Move 2 : Building on previous research
　☐ Step 1 : Findings of previous research
　☐ Step 2 : Research gap
☐ Move 3 : Explanation of key terms/concepts
☐ Move 4 : Research objectives

左ページに示したのは，§3・2 C の Slide (5)：Objectives (p.60) に対応するスクリプトです．

このスクリプトを Move に分けてみましょう．

タスク
3・3

Move analysis：スライド(5)

Move pattern を参考にして，スクリプトを Move と Step に分けましょう．使用した Move/Step にチェックマークを入れましょう．p.143 に模範解答があります．

3・4 スピーキング
話し方のスキルを身につける

Speaking

A Prosody

 前節では Background & purpose セクションで話すことがらを学びましたね.
ここでは, 効果的な話し方を練習しましょう.

Task 3・4 **Video lesson**

 video 6
Task 3・4

Watch the video and follow the directions.

(1) Write down what you noticed.

(2), (3), (4) Listen to the recording and mark the following: pause, stress, and emphasis.

Good morning everyone, / and thank you for attending my presentation today. My name is Jo Spud, and I work at the laboratory of food science at Taters University. My main area of research is food chemistry. Today, I would like to show you how our team can use potatoes to illustrate the important process of osmosis and determine the salt concentration inside different types of potatoes. Our experiment can provide information on which potato crop is best to grow in high salt areas.

Task 3・5 **Practice with the video**

 video 7
Task 3・5

Watch the video and practice speaking paying attention to the skills you learned.

Task 3・6 **Watch the video**

 video 8
Task 3・6

Compare the two presentations. How are they different?

ここでは，Unit 1 で紹介したプロソディを復習し，実践しましょう．プロソディの3原則を覚えていますか？

えーっと，1つ目は chunk ごとに区切りを入れる，2つ目は英語らしいリズムにするために stress を置く，そして3つ目はキーワードやキーフレーズを強調して発音するという emphasis です．

 そのとおり！

でも実践するのは難しいんですよね．

 繰返し練習するとよいでしょう．video 6 にある Humpty Dumpty や DNA の構造の論文の冒頭部分の音声を真似してみてください．Stress を置くところで手で膝をたたくとラップミュージックの感覚で練習できますよ！

やってみると楽しいですね！

ポイント プロソディの復習

上手な発表者:
- 文を意味のかたまり（chunk）ごとに区切る
- 内容語に強勢（stress）を置くことによって英語らしいリズムをつける
- 重要なポイントを強調する（emphasis）

ぎこちない発表者:
- 単語ごとにぶつぶつと区切りながら発音する，または意味のかたまりに関係なく区切る（発音が難しい・わからない単語の前で一瞬止まる）
- どの語も同じ調子で発音するので，聞いていてどの語が重要なのかわからない．抑揚がない．

タスク 3・4　　**Video lesson**　　　　　▶️ video 6

video 6 を見て，タスクに取組みましょう．

タスク 3・5　　**Practice with the video**　　　　　▶️ video 7

上で学んだスキルを活用して，video 7 を見ながらモデルに合わせ何度も練習しましょう．発音，プロソディ，話すスピードに気をつけましょう．

タスク 3・6　　**Watch the video**　　　　　▶️ video 8

video 8 を見て，2つのプレゼンテーションを比べましょう．

Background & purpose セクションについて学んだことを実践しましょう.

Task 3・7 Your presentation

Work on the background section of your own presentation. Use the following expressions.
(See "Useful expressions" on p.146)

Background & purpose section	
■ Move 1 : Transition (Outline → Background)	▸ Let's go into the main part. ▸ Now, I'd like to move on to the main part. ▸ Okay, let's go on to the main part.
■ Move 2 : Building on previous research 　　　Step 1 : Findings of previous research 　　　Step 2 : Research gap	▸ Previous studies have found that… ▸ (*Surname*) has found that… ▸ We already know that… ▸ However, little is known about…
■ Move 3 : Explanation of key terms/concepts	▸ X is defined as…
■ Move 4 : Research objectives	▸ Here you see our research questions. ▸ Our objective was to…

| タスク
3・7 | **Your presentation** |

Background & purpose セクションのスライドとスクリプトを作成しましょう. 左ページに示した表現を使うことができます. 必要に応じて, 付録A: 機能表現集 (p.146) を参照しましょう.

(1) スライドのイメージ図を書いてみよう.

(2) スクリプトを書いてみよう.

▇ Checklist

 あなたが準備したスライド，スクリプト，そして話し方について，以下のことができているか確認しましょう．

☑ Slide design

☐ Information from previous research is clearly presented.	… 先行研究の情報が明確に示されている
☐ Research gap is appropriately presented.	… これまでにわかっていないことが明確に示されている
☐ Terms that are specific to the presentation topic are defined.	… 発表のトピックに関する用語の定義がある
☐ Important ideas of the presentation topic are explained.	… 発表のトピックに関する重要な概念の説明がある
☐ The purpose of the study (research objectives) is clearly stated.	… 研究目的が明確に示されている
☐ The font type and size are appropriate.	… フォントの種類，サイズが適切である
☐ There are no unnecessary pictures or images on the slide.	… 不必要な画像を挿入していない

☑ Script

☐ The script contains appropriate moves and steps.	… 適切な Move/Step が使用されている
☐ The script follows the order of the slides.	… 話す順番がスライドの順番に沿っている
☐ The script sticks to the slide content.	… 話す内容がスライドと合っている

☑ Speaking

☐ Pauses are used properly.	… ポーズを適切に使っている
☐ Stresses are placed properly to create the rhythm of natural English.	… 強勢が適切に置かれている
☐ Emphases are made on the important ideas.	… 重要なポイントを強調している
☐ Voice is loud and clear enough to reach the audience.	… 声がはっきりと十分に聴き手に届いている

4・1 目　的
実験材料と方法の伝え方を知る

Purpose

A　Presenting materials and methods used in the research

Unit 4 では，Materials & methods セクションについて学んでいきます．
まずはこのセクションの目的をおさえましょう．

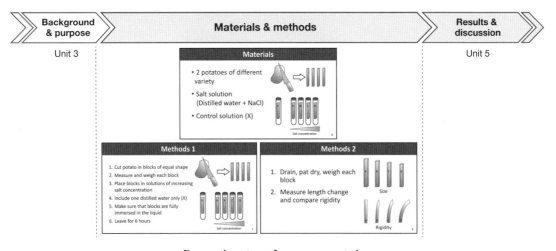

Preparation stages for your presentation

Functions

The materials and methods section describes things that were used and the study procedure.

• Fully describe the materials used in the study.
• Present the research methods in a clear and concise way.
• Follow the style of presentation of your research field.

実験材料と方法（Materials & methods）セクションの目的は何ですか？

 研究で使用した材料，研究方法をシンプルかつ明確に示すのが目的です．
2つポイントがあります．1つには研究で使用した材料を過不足なく提示すること，次に，研究方法をわかりやすく示すことです．

先日聞いたプレゼンテーションにはこのセクションはなかったです．

 いいことに気づきましたね．セクションの立て方は研究分野や研究の内容によって異なることがあります．
Results セクションで研究に使用した材料，方法，結果をまとめて発表することもあります．

セクションのよび方を Materials & methods ではなく，Methods あるいは Procedure とよぶこともあります．この教科書ではラボで行った実験報告のプレゼンテーションの仕方を紹介していますが，野外での観察や，コンピュータを使ったシミュレーションなどの場合は，セクションのよび方を適宜変えます．研究分野の一般的な発表方法にならうことが基本です．学会や研究室のプレゼンテーションを見てその特徴を把握しましょう．ただし，どの分野にも共通する英語表現は多いので，それらを積極的に学びましょう．

実験材料と方法（Materials & methods）セクションの目的
- 研究で使用した材料を過不足なく提示する
- 研究方法をわかりやすく示す
- 自分の分野の発表方法に従う

A　**Slide (6)：Materials** (materials / participants of the study)

 まず，Materials スライドに何を書いたらよいか見ていきましょう．

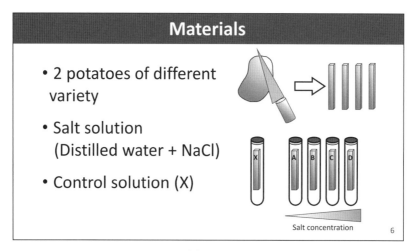

Slide (6)：Materials

Functions

- List the materials along with the steps of the methods.
- Describe the number of each material used or its quantity with figures or units.

実験材料（Materials）スライドには具体的にどのような
ものを書きますか？

 研究で用いた試料・材料は，基本的に載せます．プレゼ
ンテーションで言及しない詳細な情報は必要ありませ
ん．ただし，発表後の質疑応答の際に，質問される場合
があるので，自分のメモとして用意しておくことは重要
です．

人が実験材料に相当する場合は，何か呼び方があるので
すか？

 実験参加者（participants）という表現を使います．自ら
の意思によって研究に参加する人ということを示してい
ます．それから，実験動物のことは experimental animals
や laboratory animals といいます．

ほかに気を付けることは何ですか？

 記載する順番が，このあとで記述する実験方法の手順と
対応していること，そして，どのくらいの数や量を使用
したか，数字と単位で示すことが重要です．
また，写真を載せるときには，スケールバーを忘れない
ようにしましょう．

実験材料には，使用した機器も含まれます．当たり前の
ように使用する器具を除き，結果を得るために重要な機
器は必ず記載します．

実験材料と方法
  materials and methods
実験参加者 participants
実験動物
  experimental / laboratory animals
実験機器 laboratory equipment

ポイント Materials スライド〔スラ
イド(6)〕
● 使用した順で示す
● 使用した試料・材料の数や量は数
  字や単位で表す
● 試料・材料の写真には，スケール
  バーをつける

B | Slides (7), (8): Methods (procedure of the study / analytical methods)

次は Methods スライドのポイントを見ていきましょう.

Methods 1

1. Cut potato in blocks of equal shape
2. Measure and weigh each block
3. Place blocks in solutions of increasing salt concentration
4. Include one distilled water only (X)
5. Make sure that blocks are fully immersed in the liquid
6. Leave for 6 hours

Salt concentration

7

Slide (7): Methods 1

Methods 2

1. Drain, pat dry, weigh each block
2. Measure length change and compare rigidity

Size

Rigidity

8

Slide (8): Methods 2

Functions

• List the methods in chronological order.
• Write like a cooking recipe. Use the imperative.

Methods スライドは必ず作りますか？

 いいところに気がつきましたね．研究の種類によって変わってきます．
たとえば，研究のテーマが何かの「方法」に関することであれば，このスライドは必須です．また，特別な実験方法を用いた場合は，それを紹介する必要があります．

一方で，すでに確立された方法（プロトコル）やその分野ではよく知られた方法の場合は，結果を示すときにそれらに言及することもあります．その場合，独立した Methods スライドを作成しないこともあります．
ここでは，Methods スライドを独立して作成する場合を見ていきます．

重要な点はなんですか？

 時系列で示すということです．ほかの研究者が研究を再現できるように示す必要があります．料理のレシピのような書き方になっていることに気がつきますね．つまり，命令形を使って記載します．
この研究では実験の手順が時系列で大きく 2 つに分けられるので，2 枚のスライドに分けて提示しています．

研究方法を記述するときにほかに気を付けることはありますか？

 人や動物を研究対象にした場合，その研究対象を選択した基準や選択方法を記載することも重要です．それらの研究対象の比較研究を行う場合は，グループ分けおよびランダム化の方法を記載することも重要です．
その他，得られたデータを分析する場合は，その分析方法も記載します．

なるほど，このセクションが研究分野あるいは研究の内容によって異なるということがよくわかりました．

Vocabulary
方法論 methodology
方　法 method
実験手順 procedure
プロトコル protocol
選択基準 selection criteria
比較研究 comparative study
ランダム化 randomization
データ分析 data analysis
再現実験 replication stndy

ポイント **Methods** スライド〔スライド(7)，(8)〕
• 実験手順は時系列で書く
• 料理のレシピのように命令形を使うことが多いが，過去形で書くこともある
• 複数のスライドを使うこともある
• 再現実験ができるように具体的に書く

Preparation of script

A　Move analysis : Slide (6) to Slide (8)

> Materials & methods セクションで話すことがらを準備するために，
> まず Move 構成を確認しましょう．

Move pattern

- Move 1 : Transition (Background → Materials)
    - Step 1 : Transition
    - Step 2 : Review of the purpose
- Move 2 : Introduction of the materials
- Move 3 : Transition (Materials → Methods)
- Move 4 : Introduction of the research methods
    - Step 1 : Procedure
    - Step 2 : Comments on the procedure

Variation 1

- ◉ Move 1 : Transition (Background → Materials)
- ▪ Move 2 : Introduction of the materials
- ▪ Move 3 : Transition (Materials → Methods)
- ◉ Move 4 : Introduction of the research methods

Variation 2

- ▪ Move 1 : Transition (Background → Materials)
    - Step 1 : Transition
    - Step 2 : Review of the purpose
- ▪ Move 2 : Introduction of the materials
- ▪ Move 3 : Transition (Materials → Methods)
- ◉ Move 4 : Introduction of the research methods

Variation 3

- ▪ Move 1 : Transition (Background → Materials)
- ◉ Move 2 : Introduction of the research methods and materials
    - *Sample* : XXX was analyzed using YYY

Variation 4

- ◉ Move 1 : Transition (Background → Materials)
- ▪ Move 2 : Introduction of the materials
- ▪ Move 3 : Transition (Materials → Methods)
- ▪ Move 4 : Introduction of the research methods
    - Step 1 : Procedure
    - Step 2 : Comments on the procedure

まずはこのセクションの一般的な Move 構成の紹介です.
Move 1 は Step を 2 つに分けることができます. まず, トランジッションから始め, 次に, 研究目的の確認をします. Move 2 で実験材料や器具を紹介します. Move 3 はトランジッションです. Move 4 で実験手順を紹介します. その際, Step を 2 つに分けて, 追加の説明を加えます. これにより, その手順を強調できます.

このセクションは研究分野によって異なるということでしたが, Move にもバリエーションがありますか?

 ありますよ. バリエーション 1 は, 細かく Step に分けていません. 与えられている発表時間を考慮して, このようにすることもよくあります.

バリエーション 2 は Move 4 で手順に関して詳しい説明を追加していません.

バリエーション 3 では, 実験材料と手順・方法を合わせて 1 文で紹介しています. たとえば, "XXX was analyzed using YYY." という場合, XXX が実験材料で YYY が手順・方法ですね.

バリエーション 4 では, Move 1 で研究目的の確認をしません. このセクションに至る前に, 研究の目的が十分に聴き手に伝わっていれば, ここでわざわざ確認する必要がないと判断することもできますね.

Move 4 Step 1 と Step 2 は必要なだけ繰返してください. その際 Step 2 はすべての Step 1 につける必要はありません.

わかりました. このジャガイモを使った研究では Move 1, 2 が Materials のスライドのスクリプト, Move 3, 4 が Methods のスライドのスクリプトになりますね.

 そうです. 次項でサンプルを見ながらこのスクリプトの Move を確認していきましょう.

Move pattern
Materials & methods セクション

- Move 1: トランジッション
  (Background → Materials)
  Step 1: トランジッション
  Step 2: 研究目的の確認
- Move 2: 実験材料の紹介
- Move 3: トランジッション
  (Materials → Methods)
- Move 4: 研究方法・手順の紹介
  Step 1: 手順
  Step 2: 手順に関する説明

バリエーション 1

- Move 1: トランジッション
  (Background → Materials)
- Move 2: 実験材料の紹介
- Move 3: トランジッション
  (Materials → Methods)
- Move 4: 研究手順の紹介

バリエーション 2

- Move 1: トランジッション
  (Background → Materials)
  Step 1: トランジッション
  Step 2: 研究目的の確認
- Move 2: 実験材料の紹介
- Move 3: トランジッション
  (Materials → Methods)
- Move 4: 研究手順の紹介

バリエーション 3

- Move 1: トランジッション
  (Background → Materials)
- Move 2: 研究方法・手順と実験
  材料の紹介

バリエーション 4

- Move 1: トランジッション
  (Background → Materials)
- Move 2: 実験材料の紹介
- Move 3: トランジッション
  (Materials → Methods)
- Move 4: 研究方法・手順の紹介
  Step 1: 手順
  Step 2: 手順に関する説明

ここからは，Materials & methods セクションのスクリプトを読みながら，Move 構成を分析していきます．タスクに挑戦しましょう．

Task 4·1 **Move analysis: Slide (6)**

Divide the script into moves and steps. The first move has been indicated for you. Then, check the items you used in the "Move pattern" below.

Move 1

Next, I will show you the main steps of the experiment and provide a summary of the results we achieved. Let's look in detail at the experiment itself. / We were looking for a way to clearly visualise what happens to potato tissue when water moves in and out of it. We also needed any changes to be easy to measure. We prepared two kinds of potatoes, May Queen and Dejima. We also prepared four different concentrations of salt solutions, as well as a control solution of distilled water.

Move pattern

☑ Move 1: Transition (Background → Materials)
    ☑ Step 1: Transition
    ☐ Step 2: Review of the purpose
☐ Move 2: Introduction of the materials
☐ Move 3: Transition (Materials → Methods)
☐ Move 4: Introduction of the research methods
    ☐ Step 1: Procedure
    ☐ Step 2: Comments on the procedure

左ページに示したのは，§4・2Aの Slide (6)：Materials (p.78) に対応するスクリプトです．

このスクリプトを Move に分けてみましょう．

タスク
4・1

Move analysis： スライド (6)

Move pattern を参考にして，スクリプトを Move と Step に分けましょう．使用した Move/Step にチェックマークを入れましょう．p.143 に模範解答があります．

C | Script: Slides (7), (8) "Methods"

 前項にひきつづき，Materials & methods セクションのスクリプトを読んで，Move 構成を分析しましょう．

Task 4·2 **Move analysis: Slides (7), (8)**

Divide the script into moves and steps. Then, check the items you used in the "Move pattern" below.

The procedure we used was as follows: We started by cutting each potato in blocks 1 cm thick and all of the same length. The next step was to weigh each block to be able to monitor any change in size. After that, we placed the blocks in solutions of increasing levels of salinity, and included one control block placed in distilled water, which you can see labelled X on the screen.

After 6 hours, we removed the blocks from the solutions, and proceeded with the measurements by patting dry and weighing each potato block. As an additional test, we assessed the rigidity of the blocks by comparing how much they bent. This was not easy to measure, but was a quick way to correlate the weight changes with the amount of water that moved in or out of the potato cells: the more water moves in, the harder the block, the more water moves out, the softer the block.

Move pattern

☐ Move 1: Transition (Background → Materials)
  ☐ Step 1: Transition
  ☐ Step 2: Review of the purpose
☐ Move 2: Introduction of the materials
☐ Move 3: Transition (Materials → Methods)
☐ Move 4: Introduction of the research methods
  ☐ Step 1: Procedure
  ☐ Step 2: Comments on the procedure

左ページに示したのは，§4・2 B の Slide (7)：Methods 1，Slide (8)：Methods 2 (p.80) に対応するスクリプトです．

このスクリプトを Move に分けてみましょう．

タスク 4・2

Move analysis： スライド (7)，(8)

Move pattern を参考にして，スクリプトを Move と Step に分けましょう．使用した Move/Step にチェックマークを入れましょう．p.143 に模範解答があります．

4・4 スピーキング
話し方のスキルを身につける

Speaking

A Posture and body language

 ここでは効果的な話し方を練習しましょう. 今回のポイントは姿勢とボディーランゲージです.

Task 4・3 Video lesson

Watch the video, and follow the directions.

Write down what you noticed.

  video 9
Task 4・3

Posture

• Good examples
- Keeping a good posture, standing straight and tall.
- Facing the audience as much as possible and keeping your body open.
- Not making unnecessary movements.
- Moving forward a bit and facing the audience when you emphasize points.
• Bad examples
- Touching your face or hair frequently while speaking.
- Swaying your body side to side.
- Fidgeting, crossing your arms in front of the chest, rocking back and forth while speaking.

Body language
- Using fingers for indicating steps of a procedure.
- Pointing slides with your hand or pointer.
- Showing the size or shape of things with your hands.

まず動画を見て，比べてみましょう．

タスク
4・3

Video lesson

▶️ video 9

video 9 を見て，気づいたことをメモしましょう．

 話す際のポイントとして，姿勢（Posture）とボディーランゲージについて考えてみましょう．

 どんな姿勢が適切ですか？

 猫背にならないで聴き手のほうを向き，無駄に動かないことです．
強調したいときは，少し前に出て，聴き手を正面にして話しましょう．

 悪い例も具体的に知りたいです．

 悪い例は，緊張することによって，気がつかないうちにやってしまうことが多いですね．
聴き手に背中を向けて，スライドを見ながら話すのは避けましょう．体を左右に揺らしたり，顔や髪，洋服をやたらに触ったり，腕を組むのもやめましょう．また，脚を不自然に動かしたり，下ばかり向いて話すのも御法度です．
心当たりはありませんか？

 あ，つい，スライドだけを見て発表してしまうかも…

 そうなると，聴き手は発表者の横顔だけをずっと見ていることになり，場合によっては，スライドが見えないということもありますね．

（次の見開きにつづく）

ポイント 姿 勢

良い例：
- 良い姿勢（猫背にならない）で聴き手のほうを向く
- 無駄に動かない
- 強調したいときは，少し前に出て，聴き手を正面にして話す

悪い例：
- 聴き手に背中を向けて，スライドを見ながら話す
- 体を左右に揺らす
- 顔や髪，洋服をやたらに触る
- 腕を組む
- 脚を不自然に動かす
- 下を向いたまま話す

ポイント ボディーランゲージ
- 順番を指で示す
- 手・ポインターでスライドを指し示す
- 大きさや形状を示す

Task 4·4 **Practice with the video**

Watch the video and practice speaking paying attention to the skills you learned.

 video 10
Task 4·4

Task 4·5 **Watch the video**

Compare the two presentations. How are they different?

 video 11
Task 4·5

発表者がずっと下を向いて，机の上に置いたスクリプトを読んでいるプレゼンテーションを見たことがあります．

 練習不足だとそうなってしまいます．髪の長い人は要注意です．聴き手に顔が見えることを意識しましょう．

ボディーランゲージはどういうときに使えばいいですか？

 たとえば，順番を 1, 2, 3 と指で示したり，手やポインターでスライドを指し示すといいですね．何かの大きさや形状を手を用いて具体的に説明するとわかりやすいときもあります．

姿勢やボディーランゲージを意識できるとかっこいいですね！

タスク 4・4   **Practice with the video**   ▶ video 10

ここで学んだスキルを活用して，video 10 を見ながらモデルに合わせ何度も練習しましょう．発音，プロソディ，話すスピードに気をつけましょう．

タスク 4・5   **Watch the video**   ▶ video 11

video 11 を見て，2 つのプレゼンテーションを比べましょう．

Materials & methods セクションについて学んだことを実践しましょう.

Task 4・6　Your presentation

Work on the materials and methods section of your own presentation. Use the following expressions. (See "Useful expressions" on p.146)

Materials & methods section

■ Move 1: Transition (Background → Materials)	‣ Now, I will move on to the materials and methods. ‣ Next, I will show you the materials we used.
■ Move 2: Introduction of the materials	‣ We prepared … ‣ Here are what we used …
■ Move 3: Transition (Materials → Methods)	‣ Now, let's move on to the procedure. ‣ Now, I'll show you how we did the experiment.
■ Move 4: Introduction of research methods 　　　Step 1: Procedure 　(Step 2: Comments on the procedure)	‣ First, … Second, … Next, … Then, … ‣ In this step, we made sure that … ‣ This step was not easy because …

Materials & methods セクションのスライドとスクリプトを作成しましょう．左ページに示した表現を使うことができます．必要に応じて，付録A: 機能表現集（p.146）を参照しましょう．

(1) スライドのイメージ図を書いてみよう．

(2) スクリプトを書いてみよう．

Checklist

あなたが準備したスライド，スクリプト，そして話し方について，以下のことができているか確認しましょう．

☑ Slide design

☐ The materials used in the study are properly listed.	… 研究で使用した実験材料が適切に記載されている
☐ The spelling and capitalization of the materials are correct.	… 実験材料が正確に書かれている（スペリング，大文字・小文字の使い方）
☐ The number of each material used or its quantity is described with figures or units.	… 使用した実験材料の数や量が数字や単位で表記されている
☐ The materials are listed along with the steps of the methods.	… 実験材料の順番は実験方法に沿って記載されている
☐ The methods are written in chronological order.	… 手順は時系列で書かれている
☐ The methods section is written in a unified manner (i.e., imperative form like a cooking recipe / past tense)	… 手順の記載方法は統一されている（料理のレシピのような命令形/過去形）
☐ The font type and size are appropriate.	… フォントの種類や大きさが適切である
☐ There are no unnecessary pictures or images on the slide.	… 不必要な画像を挿入していない

☑ Script

☐ The script contains appropriate moves and steps.	… 適切な Move/Step が使用されている
☐ The script follows the order of the slides.	… 話す順番がスライドの順番に沿っている
☐ The script sticks to the slide content.	… 話す内容がスライドと合っている

☑ Speaking

☐ Voice is loud and clear enough to reach the audience.	… 声ははっきりと十分に聴き手に届いている
☐ Presentation is given with a good posture, standing straight and tall.	… 姿勢よく，背筋を伸ばしプレゼンテーションを行っている
☐ Presentation is given facing the audience as much as possible.	… できるだけ聴き手のほうを向き，プレゼンテーションを行っている
☐ Presentation is given without unnecessary body movements.	… 不必要に動くことなくプレゼンテーションを行っている

Unit 5

Oral presentation
―Results & discussion
結果，考察とまとめ

5・1 目　的
　結果と考察を述べ，プレゼンテーションをしめくくる
　　A　Discussing the results and concluding the presentation

5・2　スライドのデザイン
　スライドに書くことを知る
　　A　Slide (9)：Results 1 (figures that show major results)
　　　　Slide (10)：Results 2 (interpretation of the results)
　　B　Slide (11)：Discussion (summary of discussion)
　　C　Slide (12)：Limitations and further research (list of limitations and future research topics)

5・3　話 す 準 備
　話すことがらを知る
　　A　Move analysis：Slide (9) to Slide (12)
　　B　Script：Slides (9), (10) "Results"
　　C　Script：Slide (11) "Discussion"
　　D　Script：Slide (12) "Limitations and further research"

5・4　スピーキング
　プレゼンテーションの練習をする
　　A　Rehearsal

5・5　実　　践
　練習をする

5・1 目　的
結果と考察を述べ，プレゼンテーションをしめくくる

Purpose

A **Discussing the results and concluding the presentation**

 Unit 5 は，口頭発表の最後のセクション，Results & discussion です．
まずはこのセクションの目的をおさえましょう．

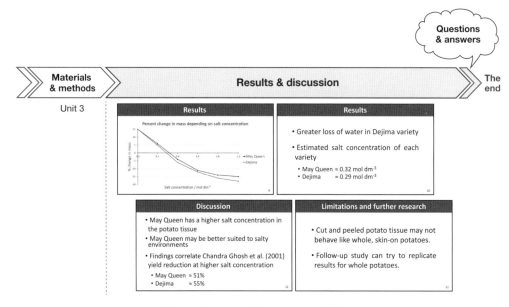

Preparation stages for your presentation

Functions

The results & discussion section presents the results, discusses the results and closes the presentation.

- Show the main results related to the research objectives.
- Discuss the results based on research objectives.
- Conclude the presentation by describing the limitations of the study and future challenges.

結果と考察（Results & discussion）セクションの目的は何ですか？

 結果を発表し，結果に基づき考察を述べ，そしてプレゼンテーションをしめくくることです．3つポイントがあります．
1つ目，最初に結果を発表しますが，その際はおもな結果だけを示します．

おもな結果ってどういう意味ですか？すべての結果を包み隠さず発表するのではないんですか？

 おもな結果とは，研究目的に沿った結果です．実験をしているとさまざまな結果が出ますが，…たとえば本研究の場合は"ジャガイモを切ってしばらくすると表面が茶色になった"などは結果ではありますが，塩分濃度の測定には関係ありません．だからこの結果をプレゼンテーションに入れていません．

なるほど！

 2つ目は，結果の考察は研究目的に沿って行うこと．
3つ目は，本研究の限界に基づいて今後どのような研究をすればよいかを提案し，研究をさらに発展させるために必要なことがらを述べます．

わかりました．研究目的に基づいて，結果を発表し考察したのち，今後の研究について展望を述べる，つまり次の研究につなげるということですね．

ポイント 結果と考察（**Results & discussion**）セクションの目的

• 研究目的に関連するおもな結果を示す
• 研究目的に基づいて結果を考察する
• 研究の限界と今後の課題を述べて，発表をしめくくる

Slide design

 Results & discussion セクションではどんなスライドが必要でしょうか？
まず，このセクション全体の流れをつかみましょう．

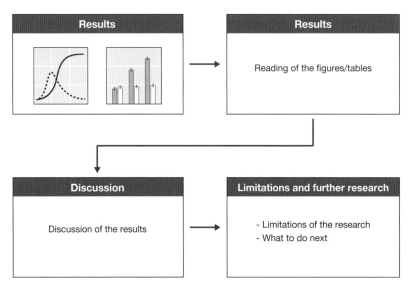

Information flow

Format

1）**Results slide**：Figures that show major results; Interpretation of the results
Give an objective description of what they represent.
2）**Discussion slide**：Summary of discussion
Provide the presenter's original analysis of the results or the presenter's opinion about the results in accordance with the research objectives.
3）**Limitations and further research slide**：The limitations of the study and suggestions for future research topics

スライドがたくさんありますね．どのスライドに何を書けばいいですか？

まず全体の流れを予習しましょう．

Results スライドには，おもな結果を示すスライドと，結果の解釈（interpretation）を示すスライドがあります．おもな結果を示すスライドには，結果だけ見やすく示します．なるべくグラフ，図や表を使い，文の使用は避けましょう．解釈のスライドにはグラフ，図や表から読み取れる内容を簡潔に載せます．

次に Discussion ですが，研究目的に沿って結果を考察します．

最後に Limitations and further research には本研究の限界と今後の研究の提案を示します．

結果の解釈と考察の違いがわかりません．

いい質問ですね．解釈は図表が示していることを客観的に表したもの，考察は，結果を，研究目的をもとに分析・検討したものです．たとえば「地球温暖化が進んでいる」という仮説のもとに過去 100 年間の東京の年間平均気温を調べ，その結果をグラフにまとめたとします．解釈としては「平均気温は年々上昇している」となり，考察は，ほかの地域の同様のデータや CO_2 の排出量などの要素を勘案したうえで，「地球温暖化は進んでいるといえる」になります．

なるほど，結果の解釈は自分で得たデータについて述べたもので，考察では，その結果とほかのデータを合わせて検討し，それを根拠として自分の考えを論理的に述べるということですね．

そうです．プレゼンテーションによっては解釈を示しながら考察を論じ，最後に Conclusion のスライドで研究全体のストーリーをまとめる場合があります．

ではそれぞれのスライドを詳しく見ていきましょう．

ポイント Results & discussion セクションのスライド構成

Results スライド:
- 研究で得られたデータを図表で示す
- データの解釈をまとめる
- データの解釈とは，図表が示すことを客観的に説明すること（事実として述べる）

Discussion スライド:
- 研究目的に基づいた考察を示す
- 考察とは，結果を分析検討し，研究目的に沿って自分の見解を述べること

Limitations and further research スライド:
- 研究の限界と今後の研究課題を示す

最初に，研究の結果を述べる Results スライドを見ていきましょう．

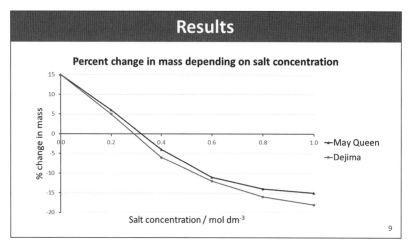

Slide (9): Results 1

Results

• Greater loss of water in Dejima variety

• Estimated salt concentration of each variety

    • May Queen ≈ 0.32 mol dm^{-3}
    • Dejima $\quad\approx 0.29$ mol dm^{-3}

10

Slide (10): Results 2

Functions

• Results are presented objectively with charts and tables.

• It is necessary to verbally state the reading of the charts and tables, but it is not necessary to have a slide solely describing the interpretation (Slide 10).

ではまず Results のスライドから説明しますね. 左を見てください.
1 (上) のスライドでは研究目的に関連する結果のみを提示します. 2 (下) のスライドで, その解釈を文にまとめて示します. それぞれを見ていきましょう.
ところで, 研究目的はなんでしたか?

えーっと, 2 種のジャガイモ (デジマとメイクイーン) の塩分濃度の違いを調べることが目的でした.

そうでしたね. 測定には osmosis (浸透圧) を使いました.
1 のスライドのグラフでは塩分濃度が $0\,\mathrm{mol\,dm^{-3}}$ から $1\,\mathrm{mol\,dm^{-3}}$ までのそれぞれのジャガイモの体積が浸透圧によって何%減ったかを示しています.

なるほど, 研究目的に直接関連するグラフですね.

そうです. そして 2 のスライドで, グラフが何を示すか, 解釈を示します.

グラフが示していることを研究目的に沿って読み取るんですね. デジマのほうがより多くの体積 (水分) を失った, そしてグラフで y 軸がゼロになる塩分濃度, つまりそれぞれの塩分濃度を文字で示しています. すべて客観的にいえることですね.

Results は客観的事実であることが大切だということがわかりましたね.

実は 2 のスライドがないプレゼンテーションもあります. その場合は図表のスライドを示しながら解釈も述べましょう.

解釈を伝えるのは必要だけどスライドはなくてもいいということですね.

ポイント Results スライド〔スライド (9), (10)〕
• 結果は図表を使って客観的に示す
• 結果の解釈を口頭で述べることは必要だが, 解釈だけを示すスライドはなくても可

先輩からのアドバイス

インパクトのあるデータは, 最後に取っておくよりも, はじめのほうにもってくることが多いように思います. 最後まで聞いてくれるかわからないので, 聴き手の興味を早めに掴みましょう.

先輩からのアドバイス

データを見せる順序は, 実際の研究の時系列どおりでなくてかまいません. 聴き手が理解しやすい順番がよいでしょう. 同じ研究でも, 聴き手に合わせて順番, 強調点などを変えて発表しましょう.

次に，研究の考察を述べる Discussion スライドを見ていきましょう.

Discussion

- May Queen has a higher salt concentration in the potato tissue
- May Queen may be better suited to salty environments
- Findings correlate Chandra Ghosh et al. (2001) yield reduction at higher salt concentration
  - May Queen ≈ 51%
  - Dejima   ≈ 55%

11

Slide (11)： Discussion

Functions

- Discussion slides should first show the results to be discussed.
- The discussion is the researcher's original viewpoint. Use hedges to avoid making assertions.
- Compare the findings with those of previous studies.

Discussion スライドには何を書きますか？

結果から導き出せる考察を箇条書き（リスト）にします．左のスライドを見てください．まず先に本研究の結果を示し，次にそれを考察します．最後に本研究の結果を先行研究と比較します．

なるほど，まず結果が示されると，聴き手は考察を聞く準備ができますね．

先行研究との比較もします．研究の結果と先行研究の結果が矛盾しないなら，先行研究の発見をさらに強化することで意義深いですし，違ったら新しい考察が生まれるのです．

ところで，それぞれの文をよく見てください．何か気づきませんか？　ヒントは動詞の部分です．

あれ？　2つ目の項目だけ動詞に法助動詞 may がついている．

よく気づきましたね！法助動詞 may を使うと断言ではなく「かもしれない」と可能性を示唆する言い方になります．
"May Queen may be better suited to salty environments" は発表者の考察なので，法助動詞 may をヘッジとして使い，断定を避けているのです．

ポイント Discussion スライド〔スライド(11)〕

• まず考察の対象となる結果を示すとよい
• 考察は，研究結果がその研究テーマにおいてどのような意味があるかを示すもので，100%確実だと断定できない場合が多いためヘッジを用いる
• ヘッジ（hedge）とは：推量の意味を加える may, might, can, could, would などの法助動詞，probably, presumably, relatively, apparently, clearly などの副詞，uncertain, probable, likely, possible などの形容詞を使って断定を避ける表現をさす
• スライドに先行研究との比較も示す

C | **Slide (12)：Limitations and further research** (list of limitations and future research topics)

 最後に，研究の限界とさらなる研究課題を述べる Limitations and further research スライドを見ていきましょう．

Limitations and further research

- Cut and peeled potato tissue may not behave like whole, skin-on potatoes.

- Follow-up study can try to replicate results for whole potatoes.

12

Slide (12)： Limitations and further research

Functions

- The slide first shows the limitations (the flaws/weaknesses of the study).
- You may connect the limitations to suggestions for further research.
- You may suggest applications of the research findings.
- Thank-you slide is not usually included in a research presentation.

Limitations and further research スライドでは研究で不十分だった点，つまり "限界" を述べたうえで，それに基づいて今後，どんな研究をすればよいかを述べます．

でも，限界を述べたらせっかくのプレゼンテーションにケチがつくようでいやだなあ…．

あはは！ 正直ですね．でもね，限界に気づくというのは大事なことですし，不足点から学ぶこともあります．それを公表することで不要な質問を避けることができます．発表者が限界を言わなければ聴き手から指摘されることになり，かえって信頼を失いかねません．限界を今後の研究課題とすればよいのです．
ただ，短い発表時間の中では，further research として今後の課題を述べるだけでもいいです．

Further research のほかに研究結果が，社会でどのように応用できるかを述べてもかまいません．この研究の場合は，ジャガイモのある品種に耐塩性があると示唆されたので，それを塩害のある畑に植えることを提案できます．

なるほど，このスライドで，自分の研究の重要性を宣伝することも可能なのですね．

あっ，そういえば，thank you のスライドっていらないんですか？

Thank you のスライドはシンポジウムなどでは見かけますが，学会発表では通常入れません．
ところで，実はこれで終わりではないのですよ．

えーっ！ まだ何かあるんですか？

はい，質疑応答があるんですよ．それについては Unit 6 (p.136) で説明しますね．まずはスクリプトを準備しましょう．

ポイント **Limitations and further research スライド〔スライド(12)〕**
- まず研究の限界を示す
- 研究の限界に基づいて今後の研究課題を示す
- 本研究の結果わかったことをどのように生かすか，その応用を示してもよい
- 研究発表では Thank you スライドは不要
- Thank you スライドではなく，研究をするにあたって協力を得た他機関の研究者の氏名や科研費などの基金を表示するスライドをつけることがある
- プレゼンテーションの中には含めないが，質問にそなえて追加でスライドを準備しておくとよい

5・3 話 す 準 備
話すことがらを知る

Preparation of script

A Move analysis: Slide ⑨ to Slide ⑫

次は，Results & discussion セクションで話すことがらを準備するために，まず Move 構成を確認しましょう．

Move pattern

- Move 1: Transition (Methods → Results)
- Move 2: Explanation of the figures
- Move 3: Transition (Explanation → Reading)
- Move 4: Data interpretation
- Move 5: Transition (Reading → Discussion)
- Move 6: Discussion on the results
    - Step 1: Findings based on the objectives
    - Step 2: Comparing the findings with those of previous studies
- Move 7: Prospects for future research
    - Step 1: Research limitations
    - Step 2: Future research
- Move 8: Ending the presentation
    - (Step 1: Thanking the audience)
    - Step 2: Asking for questions and comments

まずはこのセクションの一般的な Move の紹介です．まずトランジッションから始めます．Move 2 では図やグラフが何を示したものかを説明します（縦軸・横軸が何を示すかなど）．Move 3 はトランジッションです．Move 4 で図やグラフから読み取れる事実を述べます．

Move 5 はトランジッションで，Move 6 では，Step 1 で研究目的に基づいて，結果を考察します．Step 2 で考察と先行研究を比較します．

Move 7 は，Step 1 で本研究の限界を述べ，Step 2 でそれに基づいて研究課題を述べます．これでプレゼンテーションは終わりですが，Move 8 で質疑応答を呼びかけます．

最後に Move 8 で質疑応答を呼びかける前に謝辞を述べる場合もあるんですね．

はい，ただ謝辞といっても聴き手への礼儀として「お礼を伝える」というより，これでプレゼンテーションが終わりであることを伝えるのが目的です．ですから省略してもよいのです．

どのスライドがどの Move にあたるか整理しましょう．
Move 1-4: Results スライド
Move 5, 6: Discussion スライド
Move 7-8: Limitations and further research スライド

Results は Move 1, 2 と Move 3, 4 に分けてスライドを用意してもよいということですね．

そうです．次の項でスクリプトの Move を確認していきましょう．

- Move 1: トランジッション
  （Methods → Results）
- Move 2: 図表の説明
- Move 3: トランジッション
  （Explanation → Reading）
- Move 4: データの解釈
- Move 5: トランジッション
  （Reading → Discussion）
- Move 6: 結果の考察
  Step 1: 研究目的に応じて結果を考察
  Step 2: 自分の考察と先行研究との比較
- Move 7: 今後の展望
  Step 1: 当該の研究の限界
  Step 2: 今後の研究課題
- Move 8: 発表を終える
  （Step 1: 謝 辞）
  Step 2: 質疑応答の呼びかけ

見てみよう

今まで学んだことを意識しながら，Unit 2 で紹介した食作用についてのプレゼンテーション（中級レベル）を見直してみましょう．
Watch a presentation on phagocytosis (intermediate level).

 video 2
Presentation example
(intermediate level)

 video 12
Presentation example
(intermediate level)
Japanese ver.

B Script: Slides (9), (10) "Results"

 ここからは，Results & discussion セクションのスクリプトを読みながら Move 構成を具体的に分析していきます．タスクに挑戦しましょう．

Task 5·1 Move analysis: Slides (9), (10)

Divide the script into moves and steps. The first move has been indicated for you. Then, check the items you used in the "Move pattern" below.

Move 1

Using this method, we got the following results: / As you can see from the chart, there was a significant change in mass that clearly correlated with the change in salinity. In distilled water, and at very low salt concentrations, the potato absorbed water through osmosis, and the weight increased, which you can see on the left side of the chart. At higher salt concentrations, water went from the less concentrated potato into the solution resulting in a decrease in weight. The spot where the line crosses the *y*-axis is the isotonic equilibrium where the concentration is the same on both sides of the membrane.

Let me now turn to the actual data. The chart indicates that Dejima samples lost more water than May Queen samples. The spot where there is no change in mass is the isotonic equilibrium where salt concentration is the same on both sides of the membrane. From this point we could estimate the salt concentration of each potato variety to be around 0.32 mol dm^{-3} for the May Queen, and 0.29 mol dm^{-3} for Dejima.

Move pattern

☑ Move 1: Transition (Methods → Results)
☐ Move 2: Explanation of the figures
☐ Move 3: Transition (Explanation → Reading)
☐ Move 4: Data interpretation
☐ Move 5: Transition (Reading → Discussion)
(Continued on the next page.)

☐ Move 6: Discussion on the results
　　☐ Step 1: Findings based on the objectives
　　☐ Step 2: Comparing the findings with those of previous studies
☐ Move 7: Prospects for future research
　　☐ Step 1: Research limitations
　　☐ Step 2: Future research
☐ Move 8: Ending the presentation
　　☐ (Step 1: Thanking the audience)
　　☐ Step 2: Asking for questions and comments

左ページに示したのは，§5・2Aの Slide（9）: Results 1,
Slide（10）: Results 2（p.100）に対応するスクリプトで
す．

このスクリプトを Move に分けてみましょう．

**タスク
5・1**　　　**Move analysis: スライド(9), (10)**

Move pattern を参考にして，スクリプトを Move と Step に分けてみよう．使用した Move/Step
にチェックマークを入れましょう．p.143 に模範解答があります．

前項にひきつづき，Results & discussion セクションのスクリプトを読んで，Move 構成を分析しましょう．

Task 5・2 **Move analysis：Slide (11)**

Divide the script into moves and steps. Then, check the items you used in the "Move pattern" below.

These results suggest that the May Queen variety of potato has a slightly higher salt concentration, and should therefore be more tolerant of environments with more salty soils. Our findings match the results of Chandra Ghosh, Asanuma, Kusutani and Toyota who measured that the Dejima variety produces a lower yield overall under salt stress conditions.

Move pattern

☐ Move 1：Transition (Methods → Results)
☐ Move 2：Explanation of the figures
☐ Move 3：Transition (Explanation → Reading)
☐ Move 4：Data interpretation
☐ Move 5：Transition (Reading → Discussion)
☐ Move 6：Discussion on the results
　　☐ Step 1：Findings based on the objectives
　　☐ Step 2：Comparing the findings with those of previous studies
☐ Move 7：Prospects for future research
　　☐ Step 1：Research limitations
　　☐ Step 2：Future research
☐ Move 8：Ending the presentation
　　☐ (Step 1：Thanking the audience)
　　☐ Step 2：Asking for questions and comments

左ページに示したのは，§5・2Bの Slide (11)：Discussion (p.102) に対応するスクリプトです．

このスクリプトを Move に分けてみましょう．

タスク 5・2　**Move analysis：スライド (11)**

Move pattern を参考にして，スクリプトを Move と Step に分けましょう．使用した Move/Step にチェックマークを入れましょう．p.143 に模範解答があります．

最後に Move 8 Step 1 の謝辞を述べるとしたらどんな風に述べますか？

このあと質疑応答がありますから，謝辞を述べるとしても "Thank you." と一言でいいです．
"Thank you for your listening." と言う人がいますが，"your" をつけるのはおかしいです．正しくは "Thank you for listening." です．

Tips　**Move 8**
謝辞の代わりにシンプルに "This is the end of my presentation. Any questions?" のように言うこともあります．

D Script: Slide (12) "Limitations and further research"

前項にひきつづき, Results & discussion セクションのスクリプトを読んで, Move 構成を分析しましょう.

Task 5·3 Move analysis: Slide (12)

Divide the script into moves and steps. Then, check the items you used in the "Move pattern" below.

> A limitation of this study is that we tested potato tissue only, while potatoes in the ground have the skin on, and the skin membrane may limit osmosis. A follow-up study could assess the effect of osmosis on whole, uncut and unpeeled potatoes, in order to better assess if the method can be used for full crops. Further research could be undertaken to develop novel ways to select salt tolerant crop varieties.

Move pattern

☐ Move 1: Transition (Methods → Results)
☐ Move 2: Explanation of the figures
☐ Move 3: Transition (Explanation → Reading)
☐ Move 4: Data interpretation
☐ Move 5: Transition (Reading → Discussion)
☐ Move 6: Discussion on the results
    ☐ Step 1: Findings based on the objectives
    ☐ Step 2: Comparing the findings with those of previous studies
☐ Move 7: Prospects for future research
    ☐ Step 1: Research limitations
    ☐ Step 2: Future research
☐ Move 8: Ending the presentation
    ☐ (Step 1: Thanking the audience)
    ☐ Step 2: Asking for questions and comments

左ページに示したのは，§5・2Cの Slide (12)：Limitations and further research (p.104) に対応するスクリプトです．

このスクリプトを Move に分けてみましょう．

タスク 5・3 **Move analysis：スライド(12)**

Move pattern を参考にして，スクリプトを Move と Step に分けましょう．使用した Move/Step にチェックマークを入れましょう．p.143 に模範解答があります．

ここで，これまでに学んだこと（スライドデザイン，Move 構成）を意識しながら，右のプレゼンテーション例を見てみましょう．

見てみよう

メラノーマについてのプレゼンテーション（上級レベル）を見てみましょう．

Watch a presentation on melanoma (advanced level).

 video 13
Presentation example (advanced level)

 video 14
Presentation example (advanced level) Japanese ver.

5・4 スピーキング
プレゼンテーションの練習をする

Speaking

A Rehearsal

 ここでは今まで学んだことを振り返りながら，プレゼンテーションに備えてどのようにスピーキング練習をしたらよいか，手順に沿ってやってみましょう．

Task 5・4 Video lesson

Write down what you learned.

 video 15
Task 5・4

（空欄）

Preparing for a presentation

Step 1 Preparation

Step 2 Practice

- Review the checklist of Units 2 to 5.
- Preview the rubric (p.160) in the Resources.
- As you practice, take notes whenever you make mistakes or feel uncomfortable.

Step 3 Rehearsal

- Time yourself to make sure you finish the presentation within the specified time.

Step 4 Check

- Record yourself using your smart phone to make sure you use appropriate prosody.
- Rehearse in front of your friends and ask for advice and comments.
- Check the rubric and see whether you have reached the full mark.

- Practice, practice, and practice.

プレゼンテーションの練習方法を説明しましょう.

まず何から始めたらいいですか?

まず,Unit 2 から Unit 5 のチェックリストを見直しましょう.そして p.160 にあるルーブリック(評価基準)を見ましょう.そうすると注意するべきポイントがわかります.

なるほど,ポイントに気を付けながら発表練習をするのですね.ただ何度も練習すればよいというものではないのですね.

そうです.練習の途中で気づいたことはメモを取りましょう.間違いやすいところ,すらすら発音できないところなどを記録すると,部分練習ができます.

僕は緊張すると早口になるんです.

そうなる人は多いですね.適切なスピードでしゃべってみて時間がどれくらいかかるか計りましょう.たいていの場合,プレゼンテーションの時間が決まっているので,時間は必ず計りましょう.
早口かどうか,プロソディができているか,話す姿勢やボディーランゲージが適切かどうかは録画するとわかります.スマートフォンなどで録画してみましょう.

わかりました.でも人前だと思った以上に緊張します.

友達の前で練習するといいですよ.質問をしてもらったり,アドバイスをしてもらったり,おたがいのプレゼンテーションを聞きあうことをお勧めします.
最後にもう一度ルーブリックを見て,高評価になるか確認しましょう.あとは練習あるのみです.

先輩からのアドバイス

　発表練習は,毎回最初から始めるのではなく,途中から始めるのもよいでしょう.いつも最初から練習していると,最初だけスムーズで,後半の練習が不足することがあります.ど忘れして,発表の途中で言葉が出てこなくなることも起こりえます.途中からの練習をすれば,実際の発表途中で,自信をもって話せる部分が出てきて安心できるでしょう.

> **タスク 5・4**　**video lesson**　　　　　　　　▶ video 15
>
> 　video 15 を見て,わかったことをメモしましょう.

(次の見開きにつづく)

Task 5·5 **Practice with the video**

Watch the video and practice speaking paying attention to the skills you learned.

 video 16
Task 5·5

Task 5·6 **Watch the video**

Compare the results and discussion section of two presentations. How are they different?

 video 17
Task 5·6

タスク 5・5	**Practice with the video**

学んだスキルを活用して，video 16 を見ながら，モデルに合わせ何度も練習しましょう．発音，プロソディ，話すスピードに気をつけましょう．

タスク 5・6	**Watch the video**

video 17 を見て，2つのプレゼンテーションを比べましょう．

5・5 実 践
練習をする

 Results & discussion セクションについて学んだことを実践し，プレゼンテーション全体を完成させましょう．

Task 5・7 **Your presentation**

Work on the results and discussion section of your own presentation. Use the following expressions. (See "Useful expressions" on p.146)

Results & discussion section

■ Move 1: Transition (Methods → Results)	‣ Here are the results. ‣ Now, let's take a look at the results. ‣ Let me turn to the actual data.
■ Move 2: Explanation of the figures	‣ This graph describes...
■ Move 3: Transition (Explanation → Reading)	‣ Let's see what the figure tells us.
■ Move 4: Data interpretation	‣ The chart illustrates... ‣ As you can see from the chart, ... ‣ This chart clearly shows...
■ Move 5: Transition (Reading → Discussion)	‣ Let me discuss the results.
■ Move 6: Discussion on the results 　　Step 1: Findings based on the objectives 　　Step 2: Comparing the findings with 　　　　　 those of previous studies	‣ These results suggest that... ‣ It's clear from the chart that... ‣ Our findings match... ‣ Our findings were different from...
■ Move 7: Prospects for future research 　　Step 1: Research limitations 　　Step 2: Future research	‣ One of the limitations of the research is that... ‣ A limitation is that... ‣ A follow-up study could be done to... ‣ To build up on these findings, we can further study...
■ Move 8: Ending the presentation 　　(Step 1: Thanking the audience) 　　Step 2: Asking for questions and comments	‣ Thank you. ‣ Do you have any questions or comments?

Task 5・8 **Your presentation**

You have completed all the sections. Prepare for the final presentation.

Your presentation

Results & discussion セクションのスライドとスクリプトを作成しましょう. 左ページに示した表現を使うことができます. 必要に応じて, 付録 A: 機能表現集 (p.146) を参照しましょう.

(1) スライドのイメージ図を書いてみよう.

(2) スクリプトを書いてみよう.

Your presentation

これまでに作成したすべてのセクションをまとめ, プレゼンテーション全体を練習し, 発表しましょう.

Checklist

あなたが準備したスライド，スクリプト，話し方，そして質疑応答への対策について
以下のことができているか確認しましょう．

☑ Slide design

☐ The results are shown with figures, charts, or graphs.	… 結果が図表で示されている
☐ Figures, charts, or graphs are explained logically.	… 図表が示す内容が客観的に説明されている
☐ Discussion based on the research objective is presented.	… 研究目的に基づいた考察がある
☐ Discussion is made based on the interpretation of the results.	… 考察は結果の解釈に基づいている
☐ The presenter's opinion based on the interpretation of the results is given.	… 結果の解釈に基づく発表者の意見が示されている
☐ Study limitations are explained.	… 研究の限界が示されている
☐ Further research is suggested.	… 今後の研究課題が示されている
☐ The font type and size are appropriate.	… フォントの種類，サイズが適切である
☐ There are no unnecessary pictures or images.	… 不必要な画像を挿入していない

☑ Script

☐ The script contains appropriate moves and steps.	… 適切な Move/Step が使用されている
☐ Hedging expressions are used appropriately in the discussion.	… 考察で断定を避ける表現（ヘッジ）が適切に使用されている
☐ The script follows the order of the slides.	… 話す内容がスライドの順番と合っている
☐ The script sticks to the slide content.	… 話す内容がスライドと合っている

☑ Speaking

☐ Voice is loud and clear enough to reach the audience.	… 声がはっきりと十分に聴き手に届いている
☐ Eye contact is used appropriately.	… アイコンタクトを適切に使っている
☐ Presentation is given without reading slides or script.	… スライドやスクリプトを読まずに発表をしている

☑ Q and A

☐ Slides for anticipated questions are prepared for Q and A after the presentation.　　… 発表後の Q and A で質問が予想されることに関しては，スライドを用意してある

☐ Notes are prepared for anticipated questions.　　… 予想される質問に答えるためのメモを用意してある

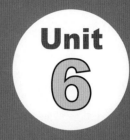

Poster presentation
ポスター発表

6・1 目　的
ポスター発表とその目的を知る

Purpose

A　Poster presentations

> Unit 6 ではポスター発表を学びます．口頭発表とはどんな違いがあるか
> まずは特徴を見ていきましょう．

A poster presentation is a formal presentation of the research, which allows:
- the presenter to use visual data.
- the presenter to explain their research individually.
- viewers to read the presenter's research on their own.
- viewers to ask questions freely.
- viewers to see a whole picture of the research at a glance.

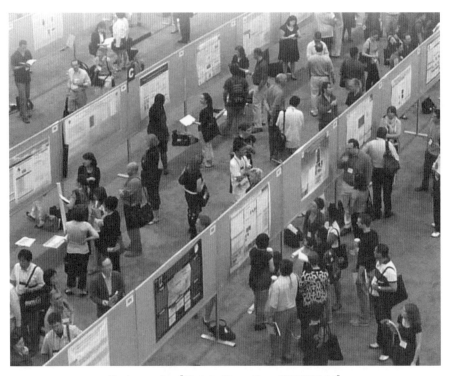

Poster session [Photo by Steven Rose, CC BY-SA 4.0]

先生，ポスター発表ってよく聞くんですが，何のことをいうんですか？

学会とか研究会などで研究成果を発表する方法のひとつで，ポスターの前で説明したり質問に答えたりするものです．

口頭発表とどう違いますか？

左の写真のように，大きな会場に研究者がそれぞれポスターを掲示し，参加者は興味のあるポスターを自由に見て周ります．発表者は自分のポスターを見に来てくれた人に対して研究の説明をします．

スライドを使う代わりにポスターを使うのですね．

ビジュアルデータを示すことは共通していますが，参加者と直接対話しながら行うポスター発表のほうが，双方向性が高いです．発表する人と聞く人の距離感がとても近く，聞いている人に合わせて説明できます．

ビジュアルデータの示し方に違いはありますか？

はい，違います．ポスター発表の場合，プレゼンター不在でポスターを展示する時間があります．そのため，ポスターだけを見て研究内容が理解できるように書く必要があります．

参加者の立場でいうと，口頭発表では口頭での説明を聞きながら順番どおりにビジュアルデータを見ていきますが，ポスターの場合は，研究成果全体を見渡すことができます．全体を理解してから，細部を確認できるというメリットがあります．

ポスターを見ただけで研究がわかるということは，ポスターに書く内容や提示方法が重要になってきますね．

そうです．このユニットではポスターの書き方や発表の仕方を学んでいきましょう．

（次の見開きにつづく）

ポイント ポスター発表とは

1) 口頭発表と同様，ビジュアルデータを活用し研究を報告する
▶ 発表者が立ち会わない展示だけの時間がある
  • 研究成果の全容を一度に示す
  • 口頭発表のスライドより説明を十分にする
  • 正確に伝わるように情報の提示方法を工夫する
2) 口頭発表と違い，参加者と直接対話する
▶ 口頭発表よりカジュアルな雰囲気
  • 服装や話し方も少しカジュアル
  • 少人数のため緊張しにくい
▶ 相手に応じて違う内容の説明ができる
  • ディスカッションができる
  • 人脈の構築に役立つ

Poster presentation and oral presentation compared

	Poster	Oral
Visuals	A large poster	A set of slides
Format	Many presentations in one big room	One presentation per room
Style	One-to-one, or one-to-few communication	One-to-many communication
Formality	Casual	More formal
Nervousness	Less stressful	Stressful
Preparations	A lot of work needs to be done at least a week before the presentation day. Modifications on the poster can only be done before printing.	Modifications on the slides can be made just before the presentation.
Communication skills	Essential	Important
Asking questions	Anyone can ask questions freely.	A limited number of participants can ask questions.
English language skills	Lack of language skills can be compensated through interactions.	A lot of oral practice is required before a presentation.

Preparation stages:

1) Plan your presentation.
- Check the data and time of the presentation.
- Check the poster size requirement.

2) Prepare contents. (p.128)
- Gather information.
- Arrange information in a hierarchical order.
- Prepare graphics (graphs, charts, tables, photos, etc.).

3) Design the poster. (p.132)
- Develop a layout.
- Select fonts.
- Choose color combination.
- Choose graphics.

4) Print the poster.
- Find a printing service.
- Choose appropriate paper.

5) Practice the presentation. (p.134)
- Practice explaining the poster.
- Practice Q and A.

ポスター発表の場合，口頭発表と違って聞いてくれる人の数は限られますね．

そうですね．ポスターの前に立って説明する時間は限られているので，大きな会場での口頭発表と比べれば，一度に聞いてくれる人の数は限られます．でも，ポスターセッションの時間は口頭発表よりも長く設定されているので，より多くの人に研究を知ってもらうことも可能です．

なんだかまだイメージが湧きません．実際のポスター発表はどんなふうに行われるんですか？

学会によって異なりますが，大きな学会では，広い部屋が会場として使われます．整然と並べられたパネルに規定の大きさのポスターが展示されます．発表者は決められた時間帯にポスターの横に立ち，関心を示してくれた人と質疑応答をします．それがディスカッションに発展することもあります．

ポスター発表をする人は若手研究者や大学院生が多いんですか？

分野によりますが，大学院生が最初に行う発表はポスター発表が多いようです．ポスターだと人脈づくりにもなりますし，大勢の聴き手の前で話すこともないので，口頭発表ほど緊張しないですみます．でも，質的なことに関しては，どちらがよりよいとは一概にはいえないでしょう．実際，発表を申し込む際に口頭発表を選んでも，主催者側からポスターでの発表を提案されたり，直前に口頭発表に変更になったりすることもあります．

なんだかポスター発表のほうがカジュアルで気楽にできるような気がしてきました．でも，英語での発表になると英会話の力が必要ですね．

そうですね．口頭発表のあとの質疑応答と比べれば緊張感は少ないかもしれませんが，質問を理解して適切に答えることが重要です．普段から英語での質疑応答に慣れておきましょう．

ポイント ポスター発表の準備

1) 計画する
   - 発表の日程を確認する
   - ポスターサイズを確認する
2) 内容を準備する（p.128）
   - 必要な情報を集める
   - 情報の配列を決める
   - ビジュアルデータをまとめる（グラフ，図，表，写真など）
3) ポスターを作る（p.132）
   - レイアウトを決める
   - フォントを選ぶ
   - 配色を決める
   - ビジュアルデータを選択する
4) ポスターを印刷する
   - どこで印刷するか決める
   - 適切な紙質を選ぶ
5) 発表の練習をする（p.134）
   - ポスターの説明の練習をする
   - 質疑応答に備える

Poster design

A　Planning a poster presentation

 ここでは，ポスターの作り方や，書くべきことがらを確認していきましょう．

1）**Audience**
- Who will view your poster?
- What do you want to tell your audience?

2）**Preparation**
- Gather your materials, and list all things you want to include.
  - Keep it simple.
  - Develop an information hierarchy.
  - Think visually.

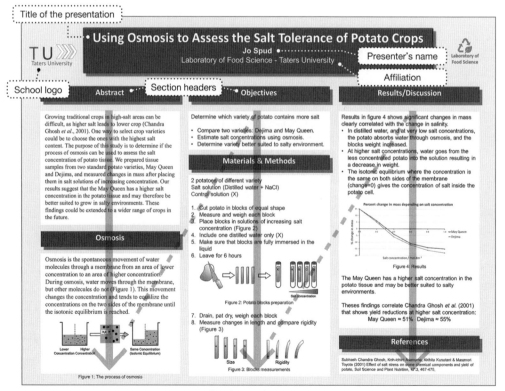

Landscape format

ところで実際のポスターってどのくらいの大きさなんですか？

小さいものでは A1（594 mm×841 mm）くらいで，大きいものになると B0（1030 mm×1456 mm）より大きい場合もあります．縦長（portrait）にする場合と横長（landscape）にする場合もあります．

ポスターのサイズは何を基準に決めますか？

会場の設定によります．会場のパネルのサイズを事前に確認しておきましょう．

大学の廊下でポスターを見かけるんですが，ひょっとしてポスター発表に使ったものが展示してあるんですか？

おそらくそうだと思います．研究室の研究内容がわかるので，再利用するのはいい考えですね．

紙のサイズは大きいですが，限られたスペースで研究成果を全部書くのは大変そうですね．写真とかグラフとかのビジュアルデータも載せていいんですよね．

もちろんです．参考資料が送付できるように E-mail アドレスを書いたり，最近では QR コードを貼って他のデータにアクセスできるようにしたりする工夫をする人もいます．

大きなポスターはどうやって作るんですか？ そんな大きなプリンターは，見たことがありません．

大きなプリンターがある学校や研究室ならそこで印刷できますが，ない場合は専門の印刷業者や街のコピーサービス専門店に依頼することができます．その場合は，印刷されるまでに時間がかかるので準備を早めに行うのが重要です．

（次の見開きにつづく）

ポイント 計 画（planning）

聴き手について考える
- ポスターを見るのは誰ですか？
- 何を伝えたいですか？

準備を始める
- ポスターに載せる材料を集めましょう
- 伝えたい内容をすべてリストアップしましょう
  - ・短くまとめる
  - ・階層構造にする
  - ・視覚的に考える

Molecular characterization of protein Y in BRAF inhibitor-treated melanoma cells

Hana Hirayama
Laboratory of Cell Biology, Horinouchi University

Abstract

Melanoma is the most aggressive skin cancer. Since most melanoma patients carry active mutations in *BRAF* gene, the BRAF inhibitor is effective in treating those types of melanoma. However, drug resistance eventually develops. A membrane glycoprotein Y is known to be a stage-specific melanoma antigen. Here, we found that BRAF inhibitor-resistant melanoma cells express lower levels of protein Y compared with those in parental cells. Resistant cells expressed protein Y species with higher molecular masses. BRAF inhibitor-treatment of parental cells led to expression of higher molecular species of protein Y and transport the variant to plasma membranes. Our study suggested that BRAF inhibitor-treatment caused alteration in molecular characteristics of protein Y in melanoma cells.

Introduction

Malignant melanoma

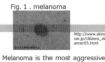
Fig. 1 . melanoma

http://www.skincancer.jp/citizens_skincancer05.html

· Melanoma is the most aggressive skin cancer.

· About 60% of melanoma patients carry active mutations in *BRAF* gene.

· After BRAF inhibitor treatments, the melanoma eventually recurs.

Melanoma marker protein Y

A membrane associated-glycoprotein Y reported as a stage-specific melanoma antigen

Y regulates migration, proliferation and differentiation of melanoma cells
Ref. ZZZ D et al. 2008

Human melanoma cell lines

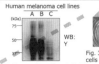
WB: Y

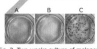
Fig. 3. Two weeks culture of melanoma cells in the presence of BRAF inhibitor

Fig. 2. Expression of protein Y in melanoma cells

C cell lines, which express lower levels of protein Y, exhibited BRAF inhibitor resistance.

Aim

To reveal molecular characteristics of protein Y in BRAF inhibitor-treated melanoma cells

Results

1. BRAF inhibitor-resistant C cells express protein Y species with higher molecular masses

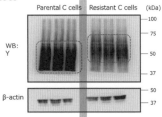

Parental C cells   Resistant C cells   (kDa)

WB: Y

β-actin

Fig. 4. The protein levels of Y in the parental and the cognate BRAF inhibitor-resistant melanoma cells were analyzed by western blotting. β-actin was used as a loading control. The signals of protein Y in parental cells were much stronger than those in resistant cells, suggesting resistant cells express lower levels of protein Y compared with those in parental cells. Since the protein Y could be heavily glycosylated, the bands showed smear. Nonetheless, average molecular masses of the protein Y in resistant cells were much higher than those in parental cells.

2. Average molecular masses of protein Y increased by BRAF inhibitor treatment of parental cells

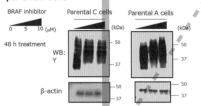

BRAF inhibitor   Parental C cells   Parental A cells
0   5   10 (μM)

48 h treatment

WB: Y

β-actin

Fig. 5. Parental melanoma cells C and A were treated with BRAF inhibitor or vehicle control for 48 h. Total cell lysates were prepared and subjected to western blot analysis for protein Y (top panels) and β-actin (lower panels). BRAF inhibitor treatments led to increases in average molecular masses of protein Y in 2 parental cell lines. These data suggest that protein Y species with higher molecular masses in resistant cells were induced by the BRAF inhibitor treatment.

3. Upon the BRAF inhibitor treatment, protein Y relocated to cell surface

Parental C cells

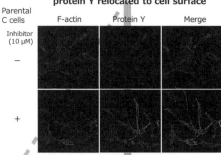

Inhibitor (10 μM)   F-actin   Protein Y   Merge

−

+

Fig. 6. To detect cell surface localization of protein Y in parental C cells in the absence or presence of BRAF inhibitor, cells were stained with anti protein Y antibody without permeabilization. Images were collected by the laser confocal microscopy. Dot-like staining of protein Y on cell surface were detected on the parental C cells in the absence of the inhibitor. Upon the inhibitor treatment, staining intensity of protein Y were markedly increased and the signals were detected at the cell periphery. This shows the inhibitor treatment also affected the cellular localization of protein Y.

Conclusions

· BRAF inhibitor-resistant melanoma cells express protein Y species with higher molecular masses (Fig.4).

· Resistant cells express lower levels of protein Y compared with those in parental cells (Fig. 4).

· BRAF inhibitor treatment of parental cells led to expression of higher molecular species of protein Y (Fig. 5) and transport the variant to plasma membranes (Fig. 6).

Acknowledgements

a Grant-in-Aid for Scientific Research (C)

Portrait format

ポスターはパソコンで作ると思うのですが，ポスター用のソフトってあるんですか？

 プロが使う DTP（デスクトップパブリッシング）のソフトでポスターが作れますが，値段が高いので学生はプレゼン用のソフトを使って作ってしまう場合が多いでしょう．化学の構造式が使われる場合は，化学用の描画ソフトを使うこともあるでしょう．画像を貼ったりフレームを作ったりするので，画像の加工ができるソフトがあると便利です．

基本的なポスターのレイアウトについて教えてください．

 ポスター発表のときは，ポスターを貼る場所があらかじめ決まっています．それに応じて基本的なレイアウトが決まります．紙を縦に使う（portrait）か，横に使う（landscape）かは，特に重要です．必ず会場の規定に従いましょう．
発表の内容を視覚的に表すために，ポスターにはいくつかのセクションがあります．内容の流れが一目で理解できるようなレイアウトが理想です．サンプルのポスター（p.128, p.130）を見てみましょう．

どこに何を書くか決まりはありますか？

 縦長のレイアウトでも横長のレイアウトでも一番上にはタイトルと名前と所属を書きましょう．書体はサンセリフ体を使います．
本体部分はブロックに分けましょう．一般的に横長の場合は縦に3つのブロックに分けることが多く，それぞれ上から下へ，左から右に見ます．縦長の場合はサイズにもよりますが，横にいくつかブロック設定する場合が多いようです．

フォントの種類やサイズはどうしますか？

 基本的に2m離れた場所から読み取れるようにしましょう．タイトル・名前・所属だけでなく，セクション見出しや箇条書き部分など，文章で示さないものはサンセリフ体を使います．文章部分はセリフ体のほうが読みやすいとされています．ポスター全体を文字で埋め尽くすようなことは避けましょう．大切なのは読みやすさです．

 先輩からのアドバイス

分野によってはすべて同じフォントで揃えたほうがよい場合があるので，専門分野の慣習に従いましょう．プレゼンテーションのスライドでも同様です．

Task 6·1 Poster design

Look at the poster and discuss with your partner.

(1) Compare the slides and scripts for oral presentation (Unit 2-Unit 5) and the content of the poster, what are the similarities?
- Diagrams
- Text
- How information is arranged
- Other pieces of information

(2) What are differences?
- Diagrams
- Text
- How information is arranged
- Other pieces of information

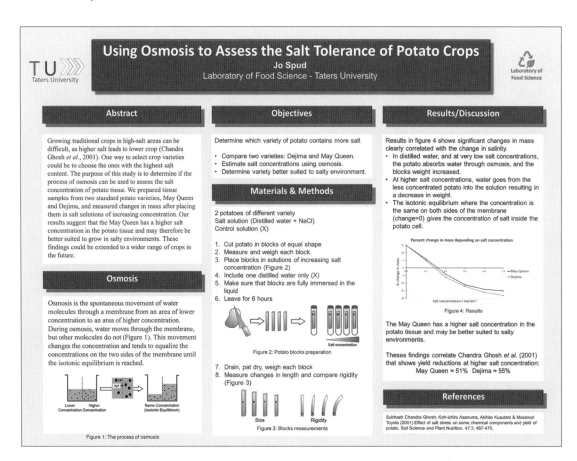

ポスターにアブストラクトは入れますか？

 アブストラクトを入れる場合と入れない場合があります．ビジュアルデータが多い場合，全体の流れがわかるようにアブストラクトを載せることがあります．ポスター自体が研究のアブストラクトだと考える場合は載せません．発表会場の指示に従いましょう．

ポスターを作成するにあたってほかに気を付けることは何ですか？

 ポスターを印刷するときは紙の質や印刷方法に選択肢があります．どんな仕上がりがよいか，考えておきましょう．ポスターは見た目が大事です．

ポスター印刷は高いので，試しに印刷する方法はありますか？

 完成したらプリンターで分割印刷をして，仕上がりを確認することができます．A4サイズの紙に何枚にも分けて印刷するイメージです．プリンターの種類や使用するソフトによって方法は違うので，使い方を調べておくといいでしょう．

ところでポスターはどうやって会場に運んだらいいですか？

 普通はポスター用の筒状のケースを使いますが，飛行機を使う場合は，折っても筋がつかない布に印刷すると移動が楽です．でも印刷するのにコストがかかるし，かなり時間の余裕をもって準備する必要があります．

やっぱり早めに準備することが重要なんですね．

タスク 6・1　**Poster design**

　左ページのポスターを見て，口頭発表のスライドとスクリプト（Unit 2〜Unit 5）と比べてみましょう．何が同じで，何が違うか，クラスメートと話し合いましょう．

Preparation before the poster session

A Flow of talk

 前節ではポスターの作り方を学びました. ここでは, ポスター発表で話すことを準備しましょう.

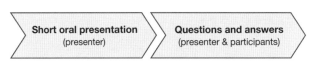

A flow of talk

A short oral presentation

- Following Unit 2 move analysis (p.40), introduce yourself and your study.
- Briefly describe your research, using moves and steps introduced in Unit 3 (p.62), Unit 4 (p.82) and Unit 5 (p.106).
- Invite questions.
- Look at the audience.

Questions and answers

• As a presenter
- List possible questions and prepare the answers in advance.
- Make sure you understand the question and the point they are asking.
- Make eye contact with the person asking the question.
- If you don't know the answer, ask if you can send the answer later by e-mail.

• As a viewer
- Look at the presenter when you ask questions.
- You can also make comments.
- If you know something about the topic, you can share it with the presenter.
- Take turns if you have a lot of questions.
- Consider others as they may have questions as well.

ポスター発表ではまず何を話したらいいですか？

 ポスターを見に来た人に，研究の概要を1分か2分ぐらいで話します．簡潔にポイントを外さず聴き手にわかるように説明します．その後，質問やコメントに対して答えましょう．

アブストラクトを口頭で言うイメージですか？

 そうです．ただ，アブストラクトのような書き言葉ではなく，相手を意識した話し言葉で，伝わるように話すことが重要です．最初の自己紹介とトピックの紹介は口頭発表と同じような感じです．Unit 2〜Unit 5で学んだ表現を組合わせて，発表の内容をまとめればよいでしょう．

口頭発表のときは7分ぐらいだったのを1分ぐらいにすればいいんですね．

 基本的にはそんな感じですが，相手の理解度や関心，あとはタイミングに応じて適宜変えられるように練習しておくといいと思います．ポスター発表の時間は限られているので，終了時刻間際に長く話すのは避けましょう．

英語での発表に関して注意すべきことはありますか？

 日本語ならできることでも英語だと難しいと思う人も多いでしょう．よくあることですが，ポスター発表の場合は，スクリプトを準備して丸暗記するのは絶対にやめましょう．丸暗記だと長さの調整が難しいからです．

じゃあ，どんな準備をしたらいいですか？

 研究の重要な点をいくつか考え，それぞれを短いセンテンスで言えるように練習しておきましょう．とっさに内容を微調整したり質問に答えるときにも使えます．発表を準備するときには，短いセンテンスで説明する練習をするといいですね．

口頭発表で使うフレーズを組合わせて使えばいいんですね．

 そうです．では，次ページでポスター発表のときに特に重要になる質疑応答の言語表現を学びましょう．

ポイント ポスターの説明
- 説明は要領よく短くまとめる
- Unit 2〜Unit 5で学んだMove/Stepを効果的に用いる
- 質問を促す

ポイント Q & A
プレゼンター：
- 質問を想定し，答えを準備しておく
- 英語の疑問文のパターンが聞きとれるように，ふだんから練習しておく
- 質問者の顔を見て答える

質問者：
- 質問だけでなくコメントでもよい
- 研究内容について知っている情報を共有してもよい
- ほかの参加者に配慮する

Tips ポスター発表の際は，自己紹介や自身の研究分野の説明は，聴き手が変わるたびに何度でもしましょう．

人間関係が構築できることはポスター発表のメリットです．自分の名前を覚えてもらいましょう．

学生の場合は手作りの名刺でもいいので持参するようにしましょう．

 先輩からのアドバイス

学会や研究会でのポスター発表では，説明の途中で質問を受けることが多いため，全体を説明するのに10分ぐらいかかることもあります．

 先輩からのアドバイス

ポスター発表のときは，紙に書いたスクリプトを読み上げるような形式はさけましょう．

B   Asking and answering questions

Useful expressions for presenters

After your short talk	
• To invite questions:	▸ Do you have any questions or comments? ▸ Any questions?
• To show appreciation for a question:	▸ Thank you for asking. ▸ Thank you, that's a good question.

When you do not understand the question	
• To ask to repeat the question:	▸ I'm sorry, would you please repeat your question? ▸ Excuse me, could you please repeat the question?
• To ask for clarification:	▸ I'm sorry I don't understand the question. Can you rephrase it? ▸ Do you mean...? ▸ Your question is.... Am I correct? ▸ Would you like me to explain...?

When you need a moment to think about the question	
• To buy some time:	▸ That's a really difficult question. Let me think about that for a second. ▸ That is an important question and I want to make sure I give you the best answer I can. Please let me think about it for now. ▸ Let me see if I can answer this.
• To avoid answering directly:	▸ Thank you for asking, but that is beyond the scope of my presentation today. ▸ That seems to be an interesting question, but I would like to focus more on... ▸ I'm sorry I can't answer that question now. That will be my next topic.
• To confirm what you have answered:	▸ Did I answer your question? ▸ Is this the answer you wanted?

Useful expressions for participants

• Compliments	▸ Thank you for your presentation. ▸ That was a very interesting talk.
• Requests	▸ Could you explain [ ] again? ▸ What does this [ ] mean? ▸ Could you send me the information?
• Questions	▸ Did you mean [ ]? ▸ I'd like to ask about [ ]? ▸ Did you use [ ]? ▸ Why did you choose this method? ▸ Who did you work with? ▸ Have you tried [ ] in your study? ▸ Have you compared [ ] with [ ]? ▸ What is your future plan?

ポスター発表の質疑応答について一番重要なことから教えて下さい.

 ポスター発表で一番重要なのは参加者との対話です. 発表する場合にはいろいろな質問を受けることを想定しておきましょう.

質問ですか… うまく答えられなかったらイヤだなあ. 不安です.

 私も質問を受けるのが大の苦手です. でも, 準備をすれば大丈夫. それに質問がくるということは聴き手が発表内容に興味がある証拠です. 喜んで受けましょう. 質問に答えることによって次の課題が見えることもあります.

まず, 発表の準備段階で, 聴き手からの質問を想定しましょう. クラスメートや研究室の仲間にポスターを見てもらい質問を考えてもらうといいでしょう. あらかじめ答えを準備することはとても重要です.
答えるときは相手の目をしっかり見て答えましょう. すぐに答えられないときは, それを相手に伝え沈黙の時間をつくらないように気をつけます.

でもそもそも質問が聞き取れなかったらどうすればいいですか？

 ポスター発表の場合は, 雑音のなかでの会話になります. 聞き取れないこともよくあります. そのような場合は聞き返せばよいのです. 妙に恐縮せず, 堂々と聞き返しましょう. 聞き返すことは恥ずかしいことではありません.

想定外の質問がきたときはどのように対処したらいいですか？

 少し考えれば答えられそうなときは, 考える時間をとって答えてもいいですが, そうじゃない場合は, 素直に答えられないと伝えるのがいいでしょう. 研究の趣旨から外れている場合は, そのように伝えればいいのです. それ以外に研究の資料がほしい, ほかに聞きたいことがたくさんあるというようなリクエストがある場合には, あらかじめ連絡先を印刷したものを準備し, 相手に渡すのもよい方法です.

 先輩からのアドバイス

　質疑応答では, 疑問詞を聞き逃さないように気をつけています. Yes/No 回答を求める質問か, How, What, Why かを聞き落とさなければ, どう返事をすべきかわかります. 聞き逃したときは, 正直に質問を繰返してほしいと言いましょう.

　難しい質問として "Isn't it 〜?" から始まる場合があります. 「はい, 〜ではありません」と答えたいときは "No, it is not 〜." と言いましょう.

 先輩からのアドバイス

　その場で答えられない質問の場合は, 後日返事をするために, 自分の名刺を渡しましょう. 相手の名刺をもらって返事を約束するのは避けたほうが無難です. 質問の内容まで記憶するのはなかなか難しいからです.

ポスター発表についてここまで学んだことを実践しましょう.

Task 6・2 Making a poster

Information you need:

1. Title: The title of your presentation is the shortest summary of your research.
2. Presenters' names: Include all the names of the people who contributed to the study.
3. Affiliation of the presenter(s): You may include the logo on top of the poster.
4. Abstract (Optional): You may include the abstract if the conference requires one.
5. Introduction section: State a brief background of your research (previous research, research gap, definitions of key terms, etc.)
6. Research objectives section: State the research questions.
7. Materials and methods section: Briefly describe materials, methods and procedures.
8. Implications / conclusions section: Describe key findings / major results and how they answer your research questions.
9. Acknowledgments (optional): List funding sources, your advisers / mentors, etc.

The design:

1. All the sections should be clearly separated.
2. Information is arranged in a meaningful way.
3. Letters are large enough to be read 2 meters away from the poster.
4. Leave enough blank spaces so that the poster does not look cluttered.
5. Choose a good color combination. Do not use too many colors.
6. Use bullet points as much as possible; avoid long texts.
7. Use sans serif fonts for headings. You can use a serif font for a longer text.
8. All the figures (graphs, diagrams, photos) are of good quality.
9. The figures are properly labeled. Add a caption for each.

Making a poster

ポスターを作成しましょう．左ページのガイドラインを見ながらポスターのイメージを書いてみ
ましょう．

Oral practice

Create your poster on your computer. Print the poster. Prepare a short script to describe your research.

(1) Write a script for a short presentation (1-2 minutes).

Brief introduction of yourself (cf., Unit 2 Move analysis)：

Background and research questions (cf., Unit 3 Move analysis)：

Methods and results (cf., Unit 4 and Unit 5 Move analysis)：

Findings (cf., Unit 5 Move analysis)：

(2) Practice your presentation with your friends. Invite questions and answer them.

Poster presentation：Checklist

> ポスター発表にのぞむ前に，あなたの準備したポスター，話すこと，質疑応答について以下のことができているか確認しましょう.

☑ Poster

☐ The title, presenters' names and affiliations are placed on top.	…	タイトル，発表者，所属が最上部に置かれている
☐ Information is presented in clearly separated sections.	…	情報は明確に分けられたセクションごとに記述されている
☐ Section headings are properly given.	…	各セクションには内容を示す見出し（ヘディング）が書かれている
☐ Sections are arranged logically and the flow of information is clear.	…	各セクションは内容に従い論理的に配置され，情報の流れが示されている
☐ Sans serif fonts are used except for running texts in a paragraph format.	…	文章以外の情報はすべてサンセリフフォントで記述されている
☐ Most information is given in bullet points.	…	情報はおもに箇条書きで書かれている
☐ The font type and size are appropriate.	…	フォントの種類，サイズが適切である
☐ The background color, the color of the frame, and the color of letters are appropriate.	…	背景の色，フレームの色，文字の色が適切である
☐ (Optional) A short abstract is placed on the top left below the title section.	…	（必要な場合のみ）アブストラクトが左上にある（タイトルなどのセクションの下）
☐ The introduction section includes the background information and research questions.	…	イントロダクションには背景の情報と研究課題が含まれている
☐ Previous studies are properly cited.	…	先行研究を適切に引用している
☐ Methods and results are clearly shown.	…	研究方法と結果が明確に示されている
☐ Diagrams are accompanied with required information (e.g., caption, legend, scale bar, etc.).	…	図表は適切な情報（キャプション，凡例，スケールバーなど）を伴っている
☐ There are no unnecessary pictures or images on the poster.	…	不必要な画像を挿入していない

☑ Speaking (A short talk in front of audience)

☐ A script for the short oral explanation is prepared and well-rehearsed.	…	短い口頭の説明のスクリプトを準備し十分に練習した
☐ The explanation follows the content of the poster.	…	話す内容がポスターの内容と合っている

☐ The talk makes use of appropriate patterns of expressions.	… 定型表現を的確に用いている
☐ Hedging expressions are used appropriately.	… 断定を避ける表現を適切に使っている
☐ Voice is loud and clear enough to reach the audience.	… 声がはっきりと十分に聴き手に届いている
☐ Eye contact is used appropriately.	… アイコンタクトを適切に使っている
☐ Talk is given without reading the poster nor script.	… ポスターやスクリプトを読まずに発表をしている

☑ Q and A

☐ Memorize fixed phrases that can be used in Q and A sessions.	… 質問と返答の基本的なパターンが使える
☐ Notes are prepared for anticipated questions.	… 予想される質問に答えるためのメモを用意してある
☐ Extra materials for anticipated questions are prepared for Q and A.	… Q and A で予想される質問に関して，さらなる資料の準備がある
☐ Prepare for questions that cannot be answered on the spot.	… 質問に答えられない場合の返答が準備してある

Move analysis の模範解答

Unit 2

Title slide

Move 1 Step 1 Good morning everyone, / Move 1 Step 2 and thank you for attending my presentation today. / Move 2 Step 1 My name Move 2 Step 2 is Jo Spud, / and I work at the laboratory of food science at Taters University. / Move 2 Step 3 My main area of research is food chemistry. / Move 3 Step 1 Today, I would like to show you how our team can use potatoes to illustrate the important process of osmosis and determine the salt Move 3 Step 2 concentration inside different types of potatoes. / Our experiment can provide information on which potato crop is best to grow in high salt areas. /

Slide (1)：Outline

Move 1 I would like to begin by sharing with you the outline of my presentation. / Move 2 Step 1 I will first give you a brief overview of the process of osmosis, and explain why it's important to know the Move 2 Step 2 salt content of different potato varieties. / Next, I will show how we used potatoes to Move 2 Step 3 demonstrate how osmosis works. / Then, I will explain how this experiment allowed us to Move 3 determine the unknown salt concentration of potatoes. / These results could help to quickly check which crops are more tolerant of higher salt concentration, as well as to develop cheaper ways to measure salinity in other things. /

Unit 3

Slide (2)： Background

Move 1 Now, we come to the main section of my presentation. I will first explain the purpose of our Move 2 Step 1 study. / Previous research has established that higher salt concentration in the soil leads to Move 2 Step 2 a decrease in potato crop production. / Getting more information about the salt concentration inside potatoes could help choose which variety is better suited to higher salt environments, as we can assume that varieties with higher salt content could be more tolerant of soils containing more salt. /

Slide (3)： Key terms/concepts

Move 3 Before I go over our experiment's methods in detail, I will give you a brief explanation of the process of osmosis. Osmosis is the spontaneous movement of water molecules through a membrane from an area of lower concentration to an area of higher concentration. During osmosis, water moves through the membrane, but other molecules do not. This results in changes in concentration on both sides of the membrane. As you can see on this diagram, the movement of water tends to equalize the concentrations on the two sides of the membrane. This is the moment of isotonic equilibrium.

Slide (4): Key terms/concepts	**Move 3** Here is an image of a plant with roots absorbing water. You can see root cells absorbing water and minerals through osmosis. Potato is a tuber of potato plant and is similar to a root. For osmosis to occur, salt concentration of potato needs to be higher than the salt concentration of the soil. Potatoes with high salt concentration can survive salty soil, and can be planted in areas near ocean. **/**
Slide (5): Objectives	**Move 4** Here is the research question. Which variety of potato contains more salt? 1. Compare two varieties: Dejima and May Queen potatoes. 2. Estimate salt concentrations using osmosis. 3. Determine which variety better suits salty environment. **/**

Unit 4

Slide (6): Materials	**Move 1 Step 1** Next, I will show you the main steps of the experiment and provide a summary of the results we achieved. Let's look in detail at the experiment itself. **/** **Move 1 Step 2** We were looking for a way to clearly visualise what happens to potato tissue when water moves in and out of it. We also needed any changes to be easy to measure. **/** **Move 2** We prepared two kinds of potatoes, May Queen and Dejima. We also prepared four different concentrations of salt solutions, as well as a control solution of distilled water. **/**
Slide (7): Methods 1	**Move 3** The procedure we used was as follows: **/** **Move 4 Step 1** We started by cutting each potato in blocks 1 cm thick and all of the same length. **/** **Move 4 Step 1** The next step was to weigh each block to be able to monitor any change in size. **/** **Move 4 Step 1** After that, we placed the blocks in solutions of increasing levels of salinity, and included one control block placed in distilled water, which you can see labelled X on the screen. **/**
Slide (8): Methods 2	**Move 4 Step 1** After 6 hours, we removed the blocks from the solutions, and proceeded with the measurements by patting dry and weighing each potato block. **/** **Move 4 Step 1** As an additional test, we assessed the rigidity of the blocks by comparing how much they bent. **/** **Move 4 Step 2** This was not easy to measure, but was a quick way to correlate the weight changes with the amount of water that moved in or out of the potato cells: the more water moves in, the harder the block, the more water moves out, the softer the block. **/**

Unit 5

Slide (9): Results 1	**Move 1** Using this method, we got the following results: **/** **Move 2** As you can see from the chart, there was a significant change in mass that clearly correlated with the change in salinity. In distilled water, and at very low salt concentrations, the potato absorbed water through osmosis, and the weight increased, which you can see on the left side of the chart. At higher salt concentrations, water went from the less concentrated potato into the solution resulting in a decrease in weight. The spot where the line crosses the y-axis is the isotonic equilibrium where the concentration is the same on both sides of the membrane. **/**
Slide (10): Results 2	**Move 3** Let me now turn to the actual data. **/** **Move 4** The chart indicates that Dejima samples lost more water than May Queen samples. The spot where there is no change in mass is the isotonic equilibrium where salt concentration is the same on both sides of the membrane. From this point we could estimate the salt concentration of each potato variety to be around 0.32 mol dm^{-3} for the May Queen, and 0.29 mol dm^{-3} for Dejima. **/**
Slide (11): Discussion*	**Move 6 Step 1** These results suggest that the May Queen variety of potato has a slightly higher salt concentration, and should therefore be more tolerant of environments with more salty soils. **/** **Move 6 Step 2** Our findings match the results of Chandra Ghosh, Asanuma, Kusutani and Toyota who measured that the Dejima variety produces a lower yield overall under salt stress conditions. **/**
Slide (12): Limitations and further research*	**Move 7 Step 1** A limitation of this study is that we tested potato tissue only, while potatoes in the ground have the skin on, and the skin membrane may limit osmosis. **/** **Move 7 Step 2** A follow-up study could assess the effect of osmosis on whole, uncut and unpeeled potatoes, in order to better assess if the method can be used for full crops. Further research could be undertaken to develop novel ways to select salt tolerant crop varieties. **/**

＊ 注: このサンプルプレゼンテーションでは，Move 5: Transition, Move 8: Ending the presentation が省略されている

付録A 機能表現集 (Useful expressions)

Unit 2～Unit 5 の Move に使用されている機能表現をまとめました.
プレゼンテーションのスクリプトを書く際に参考にしましょう.

Unit 2: Opening

Move	Step	Examples
Starter	Greetings / Welcome remarks	**Greeting and welcoming the audience** ▸ Good afternoon, ladies and gentlemen. It's an honor to have the opportunity to make a presentation. ▸ Good morning, everyone, and thank you for attending my presentation today. ▸ Good evening, everyone, and welcome to my presentation. ▸ Ladies and gentlemen, thank you for being here today. Shall we begin? (When introduced by the chairperson) ▸ Thank you for your introduction. I'm glad to have a chance to speak at this conference. ▸ Thank you very much Dr. (*chairperson's name*), for your kind introduction. I'm honored to talk about my research here at this conference.
Self introduction	Presenter's name / Affiliation / Area of research	**Introducing the presenter and his/her area of research** ▸ My name is (*presenter's name*) from (*affiliation*). ▸ I'm (*presenter's name*), and I work at (*affiliation*). ▸ My main area of research is (*area of research*). ▸ I'm [We're] specifically interested in (*area of research*). ▸ I've [We've] been working on (*area of research*) since...

(continued on the next page)

Unit 2: Opening (continued from previous page)

Move	Step	Examples
Introduction of the presentation	Presentation topic	Stating the topic of the presentation ‣ Today, I would like to show you ... ‣ In this presentation, I [am going to / would like to / will] [discuss / introduce / describe / argue / review/ propose / explore] ... ‣ In my talk today, I will give you ... ‣ I'm going to tell you about my recent study, which showed ... ‣ I'm here today to talk about ... ‣ The purpose of my presentation is to [discuss / introduce / describe / argue / review/ propose/ explore] ... ‣ What I'd like to do today is ... ‣ In this study, we decided to present ...
(**Outline**)	Outline	Outlining the presentation ‣ Let me begin with an outline of my presentation. ‣ In my talk, I would like to [start / begin] with (*topic 1*). Then, I'll talk about (*topic 2*). ‣ In this presentation, I'll first give a brief overview of (*topic 1*) and move on to (*topic 2*). Then, I'll tell you about (*topic 3*), and finally, I will have a look at (*topic 4*).
(**Significance of the research**)	Significance of the research	Highlighting significance and advantages ‣ (*a key concept*) can provide information ... ‣ One of the benefits of (*a key concept*) is ... ‣ The main advantage of (*a key concept*) is ... ‣ These are the main advantages of (*a key concept*) ‣ (*a key concept*) has numerous advantages of ... ‣ The significant benefit of using (*a key concept*) is ... ‣ (*a key concept*) contributes to ...

Unit 3: Background & purpose

Move	Step	Examples
Building on previous research	Findings of previous research	**Referring to a well-known topic** ▸ Let me start with (*a key concept*), which is widely known as… ▸ (*a key concept*) is widely known that… ▸ (*a key concept*) is commonly described as… ▸ To understand (*a key concept*) in more detail, we need to talk about… ▸ As you might know, (*a key concept*) is… **Referring to findings of previous studies** ▸ Previous research has established… ▸ The findings of (*researcher's last name*) have shown that… ▸ (*researcher's last name*) and others have shown that… ▸ In (*year of publication*), (*researcher's last name*) proved that… ▸ A study conducted by (*researcher's last name*) showed that… ▸ (*researcher's last name*)'s study clarified that… ▸ (*researcher's last name*) conducted research [into / on] the cause of… ▸ According to (*researcher's last name*), …
	Research gap	**Identifying a research gap** ▸ Getting more information about (*a key concept*) could help… ▸ Previous works have identified (*a key concept*). However, … ▸ Previous studies have shown (*a key concept*), but… ▸ [Understanding / Evaluating / Clarifying] (*a key concept*) [might / may] help us to… ▸ This kind of information would be very useful for… ▸ In order to…, we need to clarify…. ▸ It is still unclear whether… ▸ However, there remains one problem to be settled. ▸ Little work on this topic has been done.

(continued on the next page)

Move	Step	Examples
Building on previous research		‣ To the best of our knowledge, no research has been conducted... ‣ As far as I know, (*a key concept*) has never been... ‣ Previous research failed to [clarify / prove / explain / consider]... ‣ Previous research has almost exclusively focused on...
Explanation of key terms / concepts		**Defining key terms** ‣ I will give you a brief explanation of (*a key term*). ‣ (*a key term*) is defined as... ‣ (*a key term*) can be [classified / categorized / divided] [into / as]... ‣ (*a key term*) is often called... ‣ (*a key term*) is known as... ‣ (*a key term*) represents... **Giving examples** ‣ For [example / instance],... ‣ Let's look at an example. ‣ Let me give you an example. ‣ Let's say... ‣ (*a term*) such as (*example 1*) and (*example 2*)... ‣ (*a term*) is an example of...
Research obejectives		**Presenting research questions** ‣ Here [is the research question / are our research questions]. ‣ These questions guided our study. ‣ Therefore, the [aim / goal / objective / purpose] of our study was to... ‣ There are some open questions about... ‣ So, we hypothesized that... ‣ We were interested in...

(continued on the next page)

Move	Step	Examples
Research obejectives		**Highlighting the importance of the research questions** ▸ These questions are very important to ... ▸ These questions have never been addressed before because ... ▸ Critical questions associated with (*a key concept*) are ... ▸ Important open questions are whether...

Unit 4: **Materials & methods**

Move	Step	Examples
Introduction of the materials		**Explaining materials or groups of participants** ▸ The materials used in this [research / study / experiment / procedure] include ... ▸ We used (*instrument 1*) to measure .... (*instrument 2*) was then used to calculate ... ▸ We started first with ... ▸ We had [one / two / three ...] experimental groups and a control group. ▸ We had an experimental group consisting of... ▸ We assigned XXX to one of two experimental groups: (*group 1*) and (*group 2*).
Introduction of the research methods		**Referring to the method** ▸ All the data were collected by... ▸ We collected samples from ... ▸ (*a material*) was obtained [from / using] ... ▸ To explore... ▸ [My / our] method was very different from ... ▸ We recently developed (*a method*) ...

(continued on the next page)

Unit 4: **Materials & methods** (continued from previous page)

Move	Step	Examples
Introduction of the research methods	Procedure	**Explaining procedures** ‣ We first prepared ... ‣ We started by (*procedure 1*) followed by (*procedure 2*). ‣ Following (*procedure 1*), we ... ‣ We subsequently... ‣ To begin the experiment, we ... ‣ Then, we ... ‣ The next step was ... ‣ After that, we... ‣ After (*duration of time*), we ...
	Comments on the procedure	**Giving a tip for the method** ‣ In doing (*a procedure*), you need to ... ‣ During the process of (*a procedure*), you should ... ‣ While you are doing (*a procedure*), don't forget to ... ‣ It is better for (*a procedure*) to ...

Unit 5: **Results & discussion**

Move	Step	Examples
Explanation of the figures		**Make a reference to the figures** ‣ This [chart / figure / table] [illustrates / indicates]... ‣ As you can see from this [chart / figure / table], there was ... ‣ If you look at this [chart / figure / table], you can understand ... ‣ Let me now turn to the actual data.

(continued on the next page)

Move	Step	Examples
Explanation of the figures		‣ Let me show you the data. ‣ Let's take a look at the graph. ‣ What I would like to highlight in this [chart / figure / table] is ... **Explaining the figures** Bar graphs, line graphs ‣ The vertical line shows (*variable 1*), and the horizontal line represents (*variable 2*). ‣ I chose (*variable*) for the vertical line because ... Pie charts ‣ The (*color / pattern*) portion in the chart represents (*variable*). ‣ The shaded area in this chart describes (*variable*).
Data interpretation		Read the figures Bar graphs ‣ (*value 1*) is [higher / lower] than (*value 2*) by about 5%. ‣ There was a significant [increase / decrease] in the [number / amount] of ... ‣ The [number / amount] of (*variable 1*) [slightly / gradually / steadily / sharply / significantly] [increased / decreased] between (*variable 2*) and (*variable 3*). ‣ While the [number / amount] of (*variable 1*) increased, the number of (*variable 2*) decreased. ‣ The [number / amount] of (*variable*) [increased / decreased] 5% from (*value*) to (*value*). ‣ The [number / amount] of (*variable*) ranged from (*value*) to (*value*). ‣ The [number / amount] of (*variable*) reaches a peak, then forms a plateau. ‣ The [number / amount] of (*variable*) is relatively [high / low] at ...

(continued on the next page)

Move	Step	Examples
Data interpretation		**Pie charts** ▸ The majority of (*variable*) ... ▸ Nearly a half of (*variable*) ... ▸ More than three-quarters of (*variable*) ... ▸ Less than one-third of (*variable*) ... ▸ Only a small percentage of (*variable*) ... ▸ A large percentage of (*variable*) ... ▸ XXX accounts for 40% of (*variable*). ▸ XXX occupies 40% of (*variable*). ▸ More than [twice / three times] as many XXX as YYY... ▸ Not as many XXX... as YYY... **Presenting statistical results** ▸ There was a statistically significant difference between XXX and YYY. ▸ There was no statistical difference among... ▸ We used ANOVA to clarify... ▸ A paired *t*-test revealed that... ▸ Using the Chi-squared test, it was found that...
Discussion on the results	Findings based on the objectives	**Discussing the results** ▸ The point I'm trying to make is that... ▸ The way I look at this result is that... ▸ What we are discussing is... ▸ Judging from the results, ... ▸ It can be considered that... ▸ I would like you to focus on... ▸ One of the main reasons for ... [is, may be, can be] ... ▸ What these data suggest is...

(continued on the next page)

Unit 5: **Results & discussion** (continued from previous page)

Move	Step	Examples
Discussion on the results		▸ What these data seem to indicate is ...
		▸ I think that these data are ... because ...
		▸ I don't know exactly why... , but I think it may be ...
		▸ What's clear is ...
		▸ A possible explanation for... is ...
		▸ It may be reasonable to assume that ...
		▸ I believe that these data highlight ...
		▸ From this point, we could estimate ...
		▸ I was not able to find ...but I did find ...
		▸ This has two implications.
		▸ Given that..., I would say...
		▸ This gives you a clear picture of ...
		▸ This evidence seems to indicate that ...
		▸ Overall, we can say that ...
		▸ In conclusion, we can say that ...
	Comparing the findings with those of previous studies	**Highlighting similarities** ▸ Our findings match the results of (*a previous study*) ... ▸ Our findings correspond with the results from previous stdies. ▸ Similar results were shown by (*a previous study*) ... **Highlighting differences** ▸ These results go beyond previous studies because ... ▸ In comparison with previous studies, these results ... ▸ In contrast, these results make it possible to ...

(continued on the next page)

Unit 5: Results & discussion (continued from previous page)

Move	Step	Examples
Prospects for future research	Research limitations	**Clarifying limitations of the study** ▸ One of the limitations of the research is that... ▸ There are three limitations in the present study that could be addressed in future research. First,... Second,... Finally,... ▸ The findings of the present study need to be considered in light of some limitations. For example... ▸ I would like to point out that I have not... ▸ The findings of the present study are limited to... ▸ This research has concentrated only on...
	Future research	**Referring to further research** ▸ A follow-up study could assess the effect of... ▸ Further research could... ▸ Further research is necessary to... ▸ As the next step, we need... ▸ The next step in our study is... ▸ We plan to carry out further research on...
Ending the presentation	Asking for questions and comments	▸ If there are any questions, I'll be happy to answer them. ▸ Does anyone have any questions? ▸ Any questions that you might have are welcome. ▸ Do you have any comments or questions? ▸ Any questions?

Transition phrases

Move	Step	Examples
Transition		**Moving on to next topic** ‣ Now, we come to... ‣ Let's now look at the next slide which shows... ‣ Now, [let's look at / let's have a look at / take a look at / I'd like you to look at] ... ‣ The [chart / graph / figure] on the following slide shows... ‣ Now, I [want to / would like to] move on to... ‣ In the [next / next few] slide(s), ... ‣ This brings me to the next point. ‣ Before I move on to the next slide, I would like to... ‣ That's all I would like to tell you about (*topic 1*). Now let's move on to (*topic 2*).

Asking questions

	Examples
Specific question	‣ Could you tell me a little more about...? ‣ Could you explain...? ‣ Could you elaborate on...?
General question	‣ Why did you do this research? ‣ What gap did you try to fill? ‣ What is the key question of this research?

(continued on the next page)

Asking questions (continued from previous page)

	Examples
Clarification: Content	‣ Perhaps I have missed something from your talk. Would you please explain [what statistical test you used / how you analyzed the data]? ‣ I'm not sure [what/why/how]... ‣ When that [symptom / phenomenon] occurs, how long does it last? ‣ In your data, XXX seems to be slightly higher in Group A than in Group B. How do you interpret this difference? ‣ Could you please show us the figure showing...? I didn't quite understand why....
Clarification: Previous studies or known facts	‣ If I remember correctly, (*data from a previous study*). How is this related to your findings? ‣ Is your finding similar to the findings in previous studies?
Conclusion	‣ I could not follow how you reached that conclusion. Could you elaborate on that? ‣ Have you done the same experiment using a different material? Have you done the same experiment using...? ‣ Would you tell us if there were any exceptions that did not follow...? ‣ There seem to be other possible explanations for the results. Do you have an alternative hypothesis? ‣ What do you think would happen if you...? ‣ If you could reverse the conditions, what results do you think you would get? ‣ Have you considered investigating...? ‣ This is probably not your focus, but I'm interested in.... ‣ Well, this is just out of curiosity, but [why / how / what / when / which]...?

Responding to questions

	Examples
Inviting questions	▸ Now, if there are any questions, I would be pleased to answer them. ▸ Do you have any questions or comments?
Asking to clarify the question	▸ I'm sorry I don't understand the question. Can you repeat it or rephrase it? ▸ You are asking why I used statistical test A and not statistical test B. ▸ You're asking about.... ▸ You'd like to know.... ▸ Could you be more specific? ▸ Could you give an example? ▸ Your question is.... Am I correct?
Asking to repeat the question	▸ Would you please repeat your question? ▸ Would you please repeat that? ▸ I didn't quite catch that, would you mind repeating it? ▸ Excuse me, could you please repeat the question? ▸ I'm sorry, I didn't hear you. ▸ I didn't quite catch what you are asking.
Thanking for the question	▸ Thank you, that's a good point. ▸ Thank you, that's a good question.
When you need a moment to think about the question	▸ That's a really difficult question. Let me think about that for a second. ▸ I hadn't actually thought of that before. I'm going to need a minute to think about that. ▸ I would prefer to answer your questions after the session in person.

(continued on the next page)

Responding to questions (continued from previous page)

	Examples
When you don't know the answer	▸ I'm afraid I don't have that information with me. ▸ Thank you. Let me think about that and get back to you later. May I have your email address? ▸ I'm afraid I don't know the answer to your question. ▸ Interesting question. What do you think?
When the question is irrelevant	▸ Well, I think that goes beyond the scope of my [study / presentation / research]. ▸ To be honest, I think that raises a different issue. ▸ That is beyond the scope of my research. ▸ I'm afraid I'm not in a position to answer that question at the moment.
When you are not sure you answered the question	▸ Does that answer your question? ▸ Is my answer what you need? ▸ Am I answering right? ▸ Is this okay?
Avoid assertions	▸ Hopefully not. ▸ I don't think so. ▸ I don't believe so. ▸ Not quite. ▸ It depends. ▸ On the whole, yes. ▸ To some extent.

付録B ルーブリック（Rubric）

口頭発表とポスター発表の評価基準をまとめました（それぞれ日本語版と英語版があります）。
発表の前にこれらを達成しているか確認しましょう。

B1 口頭発表評価ルーブリック

評価項目		2点	3点	4点	5点	評点
あいさつ		発表の最初と最後にあいさつをしていない	発表の最初か最後のどちらかのみあいさつをしている	発表の最初と最後にあいさつをしているが、不十分である	発表の最初と最後に適切にあいさつをしている	
発表	a 発音（強勢含む）	発音・強勢が不正確である	発音・強勢が不正確なものがある	発音・強勢がおおむね正確である、十分である	発音・強勢が正確である	
	b 間の取り方	間が取られていない	不適切な間がある	間の取り方がおおむね適切である	間の取り方が適切である	
	c キーワードの強調	キーワードが強調されていない	強調されていないキーワードが多数ある	多くのキーワードが強調されている	すべてのキーワードが強調されている	
	d 声量と明確さ	声がほとんど聞こえない	声が聞き取りにくい	声量は十分だが、聞き取りにくい部分がある	声量は十分で、ほとんどすべて聞き取ることができる	
	e 話すスピード	話すスピードが速すぎる/遅すぎる	話すスピードが速い/遅い	おおむね適切なスピードで話している	適切なスピードで話している	
	f アイコンタクト	アイコンタクトをほとんど取っていない	アイコンタクトを数回取っている	最初から最後まで何度かアイコンタクトを取っている	最初から最後まで十分にアイコンタクトを取っている	
	g 姿勢	・姿勢が悪く、不必要に動いている ・まったく聴き手のほうを向いていない	・不必要な動きが頻繁に見られる ・ほとんど聴き手のほうを向いていない	・不必要な動きが稀にある ・おおむね聴き手のほうを向いている	・姿勢がよく堂々としている ・基本的に聴き手のほうを向いている	
	h ボディーランゲージ	ボディーランゲージがまったくない（直立不動）	適切なボディーランゲージが少ない	おおむね適切なボディーランゲージを使用している	適切なボディーランゲージを使用している	
	i 機能表現	機能表現が十分に使用されていない	機能表現は使用されているが適切なものが少ない	機能表現はおおむね適切に使用されている	機能表現が適切に使用されている	

分類		評価項目				
スライド	a	スライドの内容	不必要な情報ばかりのスライドが多数ある	必要な情報を示しているスライドが少ない	必要な情報はおおむねスライドで示されている	必要な情報は十分にスライドで示されている
	b	フォント	フォントの種類・色・大きさが不適切である	フォントの種類・色・大きさに不適切な部分がある	フォントの種類・色・大きさがおおむね適切である	フォントの種類・色・大きさが適切である
	c	図表	不明瞭あるいは不適切な図表が多い	不明瞭あるいは不適切な図表が用いられている	おおむね明瞭で適切な図表が用いられている	明瞭で適切な図表が用いられている
	d	正確さ	スペルおよび文法的な誤りが多い	スペルおよび文法的な誤りが含まれる	スペルおよび文法がおおむね正確である	スペルおよび文法が正確である
内容	a	研究テーマ	主題に言及していない	主題に言及しているが、わかりにくい	主題がおおむね明確に示されている	主題が明確に示されている
	b	研究テーマに関する情報量	不必要な情報が大部分を占めている	必要な情報が少ない	必要な情報がおおむね示されている	必要な情報が豊富に示されており，わかりやすい
	c	論理性	発表内容に関して具体的な根拠が示されていない	内容に関する根拠が具体的ではない	内容に関する具体的な根拠が示されているが，論理的ではない	内容に関して，論理的な説明が十分になされている
構成	a	背景と目的	背景と目的が示されていない	背景と目的が適切に示されていない	背景と目的がおおむね適切に示されている	背景と目的が適切に示されている
	b	実験材料と方法	実験材料と方法が示されていない	実験材料と方法が適切に示されていない	実験材料と方法がおおむね適切に示されている	実験材料と方法が適切に示されている
	c	結果と考察	結果と考察が示されていない	結果と考察に論理性がない	結果と考察がおおむね適切に示されている	結果と考察が適切に示されている

/100

B1 Rubric for oral presentations

Evaluation items			2 points	3 points	4 points	5 points	Score
Greeting			No greetings / No concluding remarks	Either greetings or concluding remarks	Both greetings and concluding remarks, but not appropriate	Appropriate greetings and concluding remarks	
Delivery	Pronunciation (Including Stress)	a	Very poor	Poor	Acceptable	Appropriate	
	Pause	b	No pause is given.	Some pauses are at wrong places.	Pauses are mostly appropriate.	All pauses are appropriate.	
	Emphasis on keywords	c	No emphasis is given.	Some keywords are not emphasized.	Almost all keywords are emphasized.	All keywords are appropriately emphasized.	
	Voice quality	d	Voice is too soft.	Voice is not loud enough.	Voice is loud enough but not clear.	Voice is loud and clear.	
	Pace	e	Too fast / Too slow	Fast / Slow	Mostly appropriate	Appropriate	
	Eye contact	f	Eye contact is not made at all.	Eye contact is made only a few times.	Some eye contact is made throughout.	Eye contact is made appropriately.	
	Posture	g	・Keep moving unnecessarily ・Not facing andience	・Some unnecessary moves ・Rarely facing audience	・A few unnecessary moves ・Sometimes facing audience	・Appropriate posture ・Facing audience appropriately	
	Body language	h	No body language (standing upright)	A few uses of appropriate body language	Some uses of appropriate body language	Appropriate body language	
	Functional phrases (Useful expressions)	i	No functional phrases are used.	A few functional phrases are appropriately used.	Functional phrases are used but not sufficient.	Functional phrases are appropriately used.	

Category	Item				
Slides	Slide (a)	Many slides contain unnecessary information.	A few slides contain necessary information.	Many slides contain necessary information.	All slides contain necessary information.
	Font (b)	Font choice, font size, and font color are unacceptable.	Font choice, font size, and font color are mostly inappropriate.	Font choice, font size, and font color are mostly acceptable.	Font choice, font size, and font color are appropriate.
	Diagrams (c)	Unclear or inappropriate	Mostly unclear or inappropriate	Somewhat clear and appropriate	Clear and appropriate
	Accuracy (d)	· Many misspelled words · Many grammar mistakes	· Some misspelled words · Some grammar mistakes	· A few misspelled words · A few grammar mistakes	· No misspelled words · No grammar mistakes
Content	Research theme (a)	Research theme is not mentioned.	Research theme is mentioned but not clear.	Research theme is somewhat clear.	Research theme is clearly presented.
	Amount of information (b)	A lot of irrelevant information	A small amount of relevant information	Some relevant information	Appropriate amount of relevant information
	Logic (c)	Unclear and hard to understand	Not clear enough	Clear but not logical	Clear and logical
Structure	Background and objective (a)	Background and objective are not mentioned.	Background and objective are mentioned but unclear.	Background and objective are somewhat clear.	Background and objective are appropriately mentioned.
	Materials and methods (b)	Materials and methods are not mentioned.	Materials and methods are mentioned but unclear.	Materials and methods are somewhat clear.	Materials and methods are appropriately mentioned.
	Results and discussion (c)	Results and discussion are not mentioned.	Results and discussion are not logically appropriate.	Results and discussion are somewhat clear.	Results and discussion are appropriately mentioned.

/100

B2　ポスター発表評価ルーブリック

評価項目		2点	3点	4点	5点	評点
発音（強勢含む）	a	発音・強勢が不正確である	発音・強勢が不正確なものがある	発音・強勢がおおむね正確である	発音・強勢が正確である	
間の取り方	b	間が取られていない	不適切な間がある	間の取り方がおおむね適切である	間の取り方が適切である	
キーワードの強調	c	キーワードが強調されていない	強調されていないキーワードが多数ある	多くのキーワードが強調されている	すべてのキーワードが強調されている	
声量と明確さ	d	声がほとんど聞こえない	声が聞き取りにくい	声量は十分だが、聞き取りにくい部分がある	声量は十分で、ほとんどすべて聞き取ることができる	
話すスピード	e	話すスピードが速すぎる/遅すぎる	話すスピードが速い/遅い	おおむね適切なスピードで話している	適切なスピードで話している	
アイコンタクト	f	アイコンタクトをほとんど取っていない	アイコンタクトは少ない	最初から最後まで何度かアイコンタクトを取っている	最初から最後まで十分にアイコンタクトを取っている	
姿勢	g	・姿勢が悪く、不必要に動いている ・まったく聴き手のほうを向いていない	・不必要な動きが頻繁に見られる ・ほとんど聴き手のほうを向いていない	・不必要な動きが稀にある ・おおむね聴き手のほうを向いている	・姿勢がよく堂々としている ・基本的に聴き手のほうを向いている	
ボディーランゲージ	h	ボディーランゲージがまったくない（直立不動）	適切なボディーランゲージが少ない	おおむね適切なボディーランゲージを使用している	適切なボディーランゲージを使用している	
機能表現	i	機能表現が十分に使用されていない	機能表現は使用されているが適切なものが少ない	機能表現はおおむね適切に使用されている	機能表現が適切に使用されている	
説明回答	j	発表内容に関する説明および質問に対する回答が不適切	発表内容に関する説明および質問に対する回答に不十分な点がある	発表内容おおび質問に対する回答があり補足説明を加えている	好感がもてる話し方で、発表内容に関する説明および質問に対して豊富な情報を提供し、必要に応じて適切に補足説明を行っている	

（発表）

ポスター	a	タイトル/発表者名	タイトルと発表者名が示されていない	タイトルと発表者名に不備がある	タイトルと発表者名が示されている	タイトルと発表者名がわかりやすく示されている
	b	要点	各項目における要点が示されていない	各項目における要点が示されているが、不明確でわかりづらい	各項目における要点が示されている	各項目における要点が、簡潔にわかりやすく示されている
	c	フォント	フォントの種類・色・大きさが不適切である	フォントの種類・色・大きさに不適切な部分がある	フォントの種類・色・大きさがおおむね適切である	フォントの種類・色・大きさが適切である
	d	図表	発表内容との関連が希薄である	発表内容との関連はあるが、不十分である	発表内容との関連があり、必要な情報が示されている	必要な情報をわかりやすく効果的に示している
	e	正確さ	スペルや文法の誤りが多く、理解しにくい	スペルや文法の誤りが目立つ	スペルや文法がおおむね正確である	スペルや文法が正確である
	f	研究データーに関する情報量	主題に言及していない	主題に関して必要な情報が少ない	主題に関して必要な情報がおおむね示されている	主題に関して必要な情報が豊富に示されており、わかりやすい
	g	論理性	発表内容に関して具体的な根拠が示されていない	内容に関する根拠が明確ではない	内容に関する明確な根拠が示されているが、論理性に欠ける	内容に関して、論理的な説明が十分になされている
	h	ポスターの内容	内容が整理されておらず、説明がないと理解できない	内容が十分に整理されておらず、わかりにくい箇所が目立つ	内容が整理されており、補足説明がなくてもある程度は理解できる	内容がわかりやすく整理されていて、補足説明がなくても十分に理解できる
	i	形式	形式が統一されていないため、非常に読みにくい	形式が統一されていない部分があり、読みにくい	おおむね形式が統一されており、比較的読みやすい	全体を通して適切な形式で統一されているため、非常に読みやすい
	j	引用文献	参考文献が適切に引用されていない	参考文献の多くが適切に引用されていない	参考文献がおおむね適切に引用されている	すべての参考文献が適切に引用されている

B2 Rubric for poster presentations

Evaluation items		2 points	3 points	4 points	5 points	Score
Pronunciation (Including stress)	a	Very poor	Poor	Acceptable	Appropriate	
Pause	b	No pause is given.	Some pauses are at wrong places.	Almost all pauses are appropriate.	All pauses are appropriate.	
Emphasis on keywords	c	No emphasis is given.	Some keywords are not emphasized.	Almost all keywords are emphasized.	All keywords are appropriately emphasized.	
Voice quality	d	Voice is too soft.	Voice is not loud enough.	Voice is loud enough but not clear.	Voice is loud and clear.	
Pace	e	Too fast / Too slow	Fast / Slow	Mostly appropriate	Appropriate	
Eye contact	f	Eye contact is not made at all.	Eye contact is made only a few times.	Some eye contact is made throughout.	Eye contact is made appropriately.	
Posture	g	· Too many unnecessary moves · Not facing audience	· Some unnecessary moves · Rarely facing audience	· Few unnecessary moves · Sometimes facing audience	· Appropriate posture · Facing audience appropriately	
Body language	h	No body language (Standing upright)	A few uses of appropriate body language	Some uses of appropriate body language	Appropriate body language	
Functional phrases (Useful expressions)	i	No functional phrases are used	A few functional phrases are appropriately used	Functional phrases are used but not sufficient.	Functional phrases are appropriately used.	
Narration/ Answer	j	Narration and/or answering of questions are inadequate.	Narration and/or answering of questions are somewhat inadequate.	Narration and/or answering of questions are adequate and supportive.	Narration and/or answering of questions are engaging and thorough enough.	

Delivery

Poster						/100
Title/Author	a	Title and author are absent.	Title and author contain errors.	Title and author are included.	Title and author are appropriate and clearly shown.	
Main points	b	Main points of each section are not presented	Main points of each section are not clearly presented	Main points of each section are presented	Main points of each section are concisely presented in a well-organized manner	
Font	c	Font choice, font size, and font color are unacceptable.	Font choice, font size, and font color are mostly inappropriate	Font choice, font size, and font color are mostly acceptable.	Font choice, font size, and font color are appropriate.	
Diagrams	d	Fails to support the text	Not supportive enough	Enough to support the text	Appropriate enough to enhance the text	
Accuracy	e	Many misspelled words and/or grammar mistakes hinder readability.	Misspelled words and/or grammar mistakes are noticeable.	A few misspelled words and/or grammar mistakes are found.	No misspelled words and/or grammar mistakes are present.	
Amount of information	f	A lot of irrelevant information	A small amount of relevant information	Some of relevant information	Appropriate amount of relevant information	
Logic	g	Unclear and hard to understand	Not clear enough	Clear but not logically appropriate	Logically appropriate	
Content arrangement	h	Confusing and impossible to understand the content without narration	Somewhat confusing and difficult to understand the content without narration	Possible to understand the content without narration	Well-organized and possible to sufficiently understand the content without narration	
Form	i	Cluttered and hard to read	Not visually appealing, which hinders readability	Visually appealing, which supports readability	Visually appealing, and appropriate enough to enhance readability	
References	j	All references are not properly cited.	Many references are not properly cited.	Most references are properly cited.	All references are properly cited.	

スクリプトのチェックリスト（**Script checklist**）

口頭発表の典型的な Move と Step の一覧です.（詳細は各 Unit の Move analysis を参照）
あなたのスクリプトをチェックしましょう.

✓	Move / Step

▌ Unit 2: Opening (pp. 31–50)

- ☐ **1 Starter**
- ☐   - Greetings
- ☐   - Welcome remarks
- ☐ **2 Self introduction**
- ☐   - Presenter's name
- ☐   - Affiliation
- ☐   - Area of research
- ☐ **3 Introduction of the presentation**
- ☐   - Presentation topic
- ☐   - Significance of the research
- ☐ **4 Transition** (→ Outline)
- ☐ **5 Outline**
- ☐   - Transition + Content 1, 2, 3 ...
- ☐ **6 Significance of the research**

▌ Unit 3: Background & purpose (pp. 51–74)

- ☐ **1 Transition** (→ Background)
- ☐ **2 Building on previous research**
- ☐   - Findings of previous research
- ☐   - Research gap
- ☐ **3 Explanation of key terms / concepts**
- ☐ **4 Research objectives**

✓	Move / Step

▌ Unit 4: Materials & methods (pp. 75–94)

- ☐ **1 Transition** (→ Materials)
- ☐   - Transition
- ☐   - Review of the purpose
- ☐ **2 Introduction of the materials**
- ☐ **3 Transition** (→ Methods)
- ☐ **4 Introduction of the research methods**
- ☐   - Procedure
- ☐   - Comments on the procedure

▌ Unit 5: Results & discussion (pp. 95–121)

- ☐ **1 Transition** (→ Results)
- ☐ **2 Explanation of the figures**
- ☐ **3 Transition** (→ Reading)
- ☐ **4 Data interpretation**
- ☐ **5 Transition** (→ Discussion)
- ☐ **6 Discussion on the results**
- ☐   - Findings based on the objectives
- ☐   - Comparing the findings with those of previous studies
- ☐ **7 Prospects for future research**
- ☐   - Research limitations
- ☐   - Future research
- ☐ **8 Ending the presentation**
- ☐   - (Thanking the audience)
- ☐   - Asking for questions and comments

ルーブリックを見て各項目を採点し，プレゼンテーションを評価しましょう．
コピーして点線で切り取って使いましょう．
〔PDFデータを東京化学同人ホームページ（https://www.tkd-pbl.com/）よりダウンロードできます〕

口頭発表用：付録BのB1口頭発表評価ルーブリックを見て採点しましょう（各項目5点満点）．

口頭発表評価シート（Oral presentation）　　　　　　　　　　　年　　月　　日

発表者名：（Presenter）　　　　　評価者名：（Evaluator）

あいさつ (Greeting)	発 表 (Delivery)									スライド (Slides)				内容 (Content)			構成 (Structure)		
	a	b	c	d	e	f	g	h	i	a	b	c	d	a	b	c	a	b	c

合計点（Total score）	良かった点/アドバイス（Good points / Advice）
/100	

口頭発表評価シート（Oral presentation）　　　　　　　　　　　年　　月　　日

発表者名：（Presenter）　　　　　評価者名：（Evaluator）

あいさつ (Greeting)	発 表 (Delivery)									スライド (Slides)				内容 (Content)			構成 (Structure)		
	a	b	c	d	e	f	g	h	i	a	b	c	d	a	b	c	a	b	c

合計点（Total score）	良かった点/アドバイス（Good points / Advice）
/100	

ポスター発表用：付録Bの B2 ポスター発表評価ルーブリックを見て採点しましょう（各項目5点満点）.

✂

ポスター発表評価シート（Poster presentation）　　　　　年　　月　　日

発表者名： (Presenter)										評価者名： (Evaluator)									

発　表（Delivery）										ポスター（Poster）									
a	b	c	d	e	f	g	h	i	j	a	b	c	d	e	f	g	h	i	j

合計点（Total score）	良かった点 / アドバイス（Good points / Advice）
╱100	

ポスター発表評価シート（Poster presentation）　　　　　年　　月　　日

発表者名： (Presenter)										評価者名： (Evaluator)									

発　表（Delivery）										ポスター（Poster）									
a	b	c	d	e	f	g	h	i	j	a	b	c	d	e	f	g	h	i	j

合計点（Total score）	良かった点 / アドバイス（Good points / Advice）
╱100	

付録E　プレゼンテーションメモ（**Presentation memo**）

プレゼンテーションを作成し始める前に，このメモを参考にして前提となる情報を整理しましょう．

学会・研修会・会議などに関する情報（Conference）	
名　称 (Conference)	
日　程 (Schedule)	
会　場 (Location)	
発表の日時と持ち時間 (Presentation date and time)	
想定される聴き手に関する情報（Audience）	
おもな研究分野 (Research field)	
トピックに関する知識の度合 (Knowledge level)	
おおよその人数 (Approximate number of audience)	
発表に関する情報（Presentation）	
発　表　者 (Presenter/s)	
発表者の所属 (Affiliation)	
発表の形式 (Style of the presentation)	☐ 口頭発表（Oral presentation） ☐ ポスター発表（Poster presentation） 　縦（Portrait）／横（Landscape） 　サイズ（Size）：
タイトル (Title)	

目 的 (Purpose)	
結 論 (Conclusion)	
各セクションのスライド数 (Number of slides per section)	
リハーサルで かかった時間 (Rehearsal)	1 回目 (First time)　：　　　　分 (min) 2 回目 (Second time)：　　　　分 (min)

使用機材に関する情報 (The equipment)	
使用 PC (PC used in the presentation)	持込み (Bring your own) ／ 貸出し (Equipped)
使用 PC の OS (OS of the PC)	Windows ／ Mac ／ その他 (Others)　(　　　　　　　　)
使用 PC の端子 (Connector of the PC)	HDMI ／ VGA ／ USB Type-C ／ その他 (Others)　(　　　　　　)
発表に必要なもの (Materials)	ポインター (Pointer) ／ 配布資料 (Handouts) その他 (Others)　(　　　　　　　　　　　　　　　)

メ モ 欄 (Memo)

第 1 版 第 1 刷 2023 年 4 月 17 日 発行

ライフサイエンスのための英語
Ⅱ. プレゼンテーション編

Ⓒ 2023

編 著 者	萩 原 明 子
	内 藤 麻 緒
	小 林 薫
発 行 者	住 田 六 連
発 行	株式会社 東京化学同人

東京都文京区千石 3 丁目 36-7 (〒112-0011)
電話 03-3946-5311・FAX 03-3946-5317
URL: https://www.tkd-pbl.com/

印 刷 中央印刷株式会社
製 本 株式会社 松岳社

ISBN978-4-8079-2040-2
Printed in Japan

ライフサイエンスのための
英　語
I. 基本スキル編

萩原明子・小 林　薫 編著

B5 判　184 ページ　定価 2640 円（本体 2400 円＋税）

生命科学分野を専攻とする学生を対象とし，生命科学の
トピックを扱いながら，学生が知らず知らずのうちに科
学英語の読み，書き，話すの基本スキルを修得すること
ができる教科書．音声データ付．

主要目次　Study Guide（科学英語習得のための効果的な学習法の手引
き）／Textbook（聴解，読解，文型，語彙の学習と練習問題，6 ユ
ニットよりなる）／Workbook[Textbookの各ユニットに対応した課題
（内容理解問題，応用問題，聞き取り，応答問題），科学英語の語彙
リスト]（切取り提出様式）

2023 年 4 月現在（定価は 10％税込）